Praise for *Acupuncture Today and in Ancient China*

"The book is fascinating. It gives great insights into the organ functions and also uses an interesting approach to explain the mental and emotional factors in causing disease. My students find the book indispensable."

- Brandon Fuller, Program Chair,
East West College of Natural Medicine, Sarasota, Florida.

"We have come across many books on Chinese Medicine and particularly like this book's approach of blending the Western and Chinese understanding of the organs, to make it clear that both systems describe the same organs."

- Sam Patel, Joint Principal,
The International College of Oriental Medicine, UK.

Acupuncture explained

Clearly explains how acupuncture works
and what it can treat

Fletcher Kovich, Lic.Ac.

CuriousPages Publishing
Bristol, United Kingdom

Published 2018 by CuriousPages Publishing, Bristol, United Kingdom

Updated 25 March 2020

ISBN 978 1 9164830 0 2 (paperback)
ISBN 978 1 9164830 2 6 (hardback)
ISBN 978 1 9164830 3 3 (epub)

This book does not serve as a manual on how to do acupuncture or acupressure. Such treatments, whether by needling, moxibustion, cupping or pressure, should always be performed by a qualified Chinese Medicine acupuncturist.

The cover photo shows a monastery in Meteora, Northern Greece. The area has unusual mountainous formations with ancient monasteries perched on six of the peaks, and is a UNESCO World Heritage site.

Preface

This book is a reduction of the much longer book by the same author: *Acupuncture Today and in Ancient China.*

Acupuncture Explained retains the most essential content from each of the organ chapters in *Acupuncture Today and in Ancient China*, but leaves out the more academic content, including the detailed references to the early Chinese medicine classic text, the *Nei Jing*, and the many citations on other topics. Other, full chapters are also left out, such as those on the history of Chinese medicine; the detailed analysis of the *Nei Jing* theories of metabolism; and the analysis of their other notions and theories, such as the Five phase theory. And also left out are the chapters on the scientific investigations of acupuncture and the details of the author's own cutting-edge hypothesis on how acupuncture works.

The text that remains in *Acupuncture Explained* provides a clear, easy-to-read account of what acupuncture is, how it works, and what it can treat—all expressed in terms that can be understood by today's readers. Hence, the text can be fruitfully read by any patient who wishes to understand their treatment, how it works and the thinking behind it; or read by acupuncture students who wish to quickly obtain this same overview of the subject, to complement their more detailed studies and to also understand how to explain the treatments to patients.

Contents

Chapter 1. Introduction

The earliest surviving record of Chinese acupuncture dates back more than two thousand years, in a series of ancient scripts known as the *Nei Jing*. These scripts describe the causes of illness (including mental and emotional factors) and how these affect the main organs. Once the organs become stressed, the scripts list the signs and symptoms that result. The meridians associated with each organ were also listed, and stimulating an acupuncture point (acupoint) on one of these meridians is able to correct the issue in the related organ.

In clinic today, over two thousand years later, all these same signs and symptoms are still routinely seen in patients, associated with stress (or illness) in a particular organ.

The layout of this book

The following chapters are each dedicated to particular organs, and describe the lifestyle factors (including mental and emotional) that cause stress in those organs, and list the possible signs and symptoms that this produces. The acupuncture treatment is then described, and suggestions are given on how to avoid such illnesses in the future.

Chapter 8 provides detailed case histories covering many common conditions, from diagnosis through to the outcome of the treatments; and these are referred to throughout the above organ chapters.

Finally, the index lists all the signs and symptoms and conditions mentioned in the organ chapters.

How to use this book

The book may simply be read through, to gain an overview of Chinese acupuncture, what it can treat and how the treatment works. Or when you are interested in a particular condition or simply a single sign or symptom, this could be looked up in the index, which would direct you to the pages where the organ concerned is discussed. This would indicate which organ is producing the condition, the likely cause, how the condition could be treated with acupuncture, or alternatively, lifestyle adjustments that could be made to alleviate the condition. If more than one page is listed in the index for that sign, symptom or condition, and the pages refer to different organs, you should read the other signs and symptoms listed for each of those organs, which may help to identify the main organ involved. When a *selection* of the signs and symptoms for a particular organ are present, this usually indicates that the condition is being produced by that organ.

The above approach is suggested as a guide to diagnosis, and to provide an insight into your health. If the signs or symptoms are pronounced, it would be advisable to consult a qualified practitioner of Chinese acupuncture to confirm the diagnosis and provide appropriate treatment.

Chapter 2. Pancreas and stomach

Each organ chapter describes two organs, since those organs are closely associated with one another, and are both often affected when either of the organs in that pair is affected.

In Chinese medicine, the pancreas is usually called the "spleen". This is due to a mistaken attribution of the organs in ancient times. However, the anatomical organ being referred to is the pancreas, and in this book I use the anatomically correct description (of "pancreas"), so as to avoid confusion when comparing this book's content with contemporary physiology.

In contemporary physiology, the main functions of the pancreas are that it

- produces pancreatic juice, which contains enzymes that digest carbohydrates, proteins and fats (these enable the small intestine to absorb the nutrients into the blood stream);
- secretes the hormones *insulin* and *glucagon* to control the uptake of glucose, which is the body's main fuel; and
- secrets the hormone *pancreatic polypeptide*, which is thought to produce the appetite.

The *Nei Jing* authors noticed that when the pancreas function was poor, any of the following signs and symptoms could be present. Usually, not all would be present, but only a selection. If about three are present, this would usually indicate a diagnosis of poor pancreas function.

- poor appetite (prefer to only eat small amounts);
- general weakness (and hence the tendency to avoid speaking), and feeling tired after eating;
- abdominal bloating and discomfort (particularly after eating), excess gas, frequent loose stools;
- intolerances for certain foods, such as dairy or wheat;
- poor sense of taste;
- cravings for sweet food;
- muscles of limbs are weak and soft (emaciated);
- tendency to bruise easily or have mild haemorrhages or purple spots or patches on the skin, blood in the stools, excessive menstrual flow or bleeding of the uterus;
- feeling a bearing-down sensation in the abdomen, possibly with prolapse of the anus or of internal organs such as the stomach, kidneys, uterus or bladder; and
- pain or discomfort anywhere along the pancreas or stomach meridian.

People with this condition would tend to be habitual thinkers or worriers, and all the above signs and symptoms would tend to be made worse after extended periods of heavy thinking or studying.

Facial colour and tone of voice

In chronic cases, there may be a yellow hue visible on the face, and the patient would tend to have a "singing" tone of voice, and may often hum or sing to themselves.

Examination of the tongue and pulses

A practitioner would confirm the diagnosis by examining the patient's tongue and "organ pulses".

With poor pancreas function, the tongue would usually be swollen with teeth indentations on the side.

The pulses are felt in three different positions on each wrist, each position providing information about the functioning of a different organ. This is conveyed in the quality of the pulse, rather than merely its speed; and the possible qualities could involve the width of the pulse, the firmness, or tautness, the shape of the rising and falling, the strength, the depth, and so on—with each quality indicating a particular type of malfunction in the corresponding organ.

With poor pancreas function, most of the organ pulses would have a quality known as "slippery".

Other terms used for this condition

In Chinese medicine, this condition may also be called "Spleen chi deficiency", which simply means that the function of the pancreas is poor.

In contemporary medicine, the term IBS (irritable bowel syndrome) is often used.

Treating poor pancreas function

Once diagnosed, an acupuncture point (acupoint) would be selected to strengthen the pancreas function. (When acupoints are mentioned in this book, their approximate location is given; the intention is to give the general reader an idea of approximately where on the body the acupoint is, rather than defining the location exactly.) Some typical acupoints are

- Stomach-36 (on the shin, about three inches below the knee),
- Pancreas-6[*] (about three inches above the inner ankle),
- Pancreas-3[†] (on the side of the foot, beside the big toe), and
- Bladder-20 (on the back).

---

[*] Also called Spleen-6.

[†] Also called Spleen-3.

Note that usually only a single acupoint would be used. But in acupuncture, there is often a choice of several different acupoints that could achieve the same effect; and the most appropriate one would be chosen depending on the circumstances. The above are the most commonly used acupoints to correct poor pancreas function.

When poor pancreas function has been present for some time, these acupoints tend to feel tender when pressed, due to the resonance between the pancreas and these acupoints. When one of the acupoints is stimulated, this utilizes this same resonance but in reverse, which encourages the organ to cancel out the malfunction in itself that caused the tenderness, and the organ returns to normal function. The pancreas pulse would then become much stronger (where it was previously weak) and usually change in quality.

The progress of treatment

In Western countries, acupuncture sessions tend to be given at weekly intervals initially, then the time between treatments is increased as the signs and symptoms improve. On the second visit, most patients report an improvement in some of their symptoms, which could include an improvement in their sense of taste, energy or digestion, with less bloating and tiredness after eating, or the absence of loose stools; and some even report an improvement in their ability to think, with their mind seeming more clear. After the first session, this improvement may only last for a day or two, particularly when the symptoms were present for many years. But after each successive treatment, the improvements usually last longer, until the patient remains symptom free between treatments.

Patient example
Male, aged 56. This patient had a wide range of symptoms which had built up for years, including poor appetite, feeling tired after eating, having a poor sense of taste, sweet cravings, loose stools, and he found it hard to think after midday. All these symptoms cleared after a few treatments. See the full case history on page 128.

The value of regular maintenance treatments

Once a patient's health problem has been resolved, they usually appreciate the value of good health and realize that this can be maintained by regular treatments, with the frequency being determined by the degree of stress in their life.

In the *Nei Jing*, it is said "When treatment is sought only after a disease has become fully developed... this is as if a well were dug when one is thirsty, and as if weapons were cast when the fight is on. Would this not be too late?"

Causes of poor pancreas function

This condition is widespread in developed countries, since they are "thinking" societies. Many jobs are mentally demanding, the education system itself demands intensive study over many years, and perhaps the situation of wealth itself tends to produce citizens who are prone to thinking and worrying—due to the pressures of consumerism. All this mental activity tends to impede the pancreas function.

The connection between certain thought patterns and certain organs was noticed as far back as the *Nei Jing*. At that time, the only way of accounting for such effects was the assumption that each of the main organs possessed a "soul", which produced these effects. For example, the pancreas's soul was called the *yi*, and this was thought to produce a person's "tendency to ponder".

However, a more likely explanation is that our conscious mind utilizes the logic of the abdominal organs to process our thoughts, so that the organ performs that same actions on our thoughts that it does on the substances it processes in the body. The pancreas digests food, and this digestive function can also be utilized by our mind to digest thoughts. This explanation accounts for the two-way association between the pancreas and our thoughts, such that when we overindulge in thinking, this has the same effect on the pancreas that having to constantly digest a banquet of food would have, so the pancreas becomes exhausted. And conversely, once the pancreas is exhausted, we find it very much harder to digest facts (see *Acupuncture Today and in Ancient China* for more detail).

A lack of exercise may also make it harder for the pancreas to function well. Gentle exercise after a meal aids the digestive process. But most of today's occupations demand lack of exercise, which only makes it harder for the digestive organs to work properly.

And finally, the very fact that we live in a developed society seems (paradoxically) to demand that we eat unhealthy food, making it even harder for the overworked digestive organs to extract the nourishment the body needs. The pancreas cannot cope with the demands we place on it, which causes it to produce many of the signs and symptoms listed on page 14 above.

Acupuncture highlights unhealthy lifestyle factors

Acupuncture normalizes the functions of the main organs, and at the end of a treatment session patients often comment on how relaxed they feel, and some even describe their state as euphoric. I usually tell them that what they are feeling is normal, but that normality only feels this good to them because they were so used to living in a stressed state.

This "normality" does begin to wear off in the days following the treatment, since the patient returns to their previous stresses, and responds to them in the same way. But after a few treatments, patients often make spontaneous changes to their lifestyle. It is as though the treatments make them aware of the factors in their life that detract from this "normality"—that is, the factors that encourage their organs to work in ways that do not feel right. And a patient with poor pancreas function might become less inclined to overthink, or to worry, since they can now so clearly feel how exhausting this is, or how unwell it makes them feel. And they may also start to introduce more light exercise, particularly after eating, and also changes to their diet.

Helpful changes to the diet

When a patient has poor pancreas function, it would be beneficial for them to avoid eating any of the following:

- all heavy dairy produce, such as cheese and cream;
- pork and rich meat;
- roasted peanuts (such as in peanut butter);
- concentrated juices, especially orange and tomato;
- bananas, sugar and sweeteners; and
- if the poor pancreas function is pronounced, wheat could be avoided in the early stages of treatment.

And in general all meals should be cooked and warm, and liquids should also be at body temperature or above. This is to aid the digestive process—since, when we eat raw or cold foods, the stomach and pancreas need to work harder to digest them; while if foods are cooked and warm, they can be digested more easily.

Sweet cravings

Most patients I see in clinic who have poor pancreas function describe themselves as having sweet cravings. This is because food that is naturally sweet tends to benefit the pancreas. However, in developed countries, people often satisfy this craving by eating chocolate or other foods high in refined sugar, which may provide a short term boost in energy but ultimately only weakens the pancreas further. This is because the sweetness is far too high. The remedial flavours that we crave should be taken in small doses, which have a beneficial effect; but when taken in large doses, this tends to overwhelm the organ and have a negative effect.

The following foods are naturally sweet and would all tend to have a beneficial effect (when adequately cooked):

- sweet root vegetables, such as carrot, parsnip, sweet potato, potato;
- rice, oats, millet;
- cauliflower, pumpkin, squash, string beans, broad beans, lentils, peas;
- blueberry, cherry, date, fig, grape, strawberry;
- salmon, herring, or any white fish; and
- chamomile and jasmine.

Effects on the quality of the blood

In terms of its nutritional content, the quality of the blood depends on the good function of the pancreas and stomach. This means that an exhausted pancreas would lead to a reduction in the quality of the blood, which could cause a range of signs and symptoms, including

- a pale complexion, pale lips and fingernails;
- dizziness, vertigo;
- dry stools, constipation; and
- dry skin or hair, with the skin being itchy.

And if the heart were affected by the poor quality blood, this could produce

- poor long-term memory;
- insomnia (where it was difficult to fall asleep, rather than waking during the night); and
- palpitations, anxiety.

And if the liver were affected, this could produce

- numbness or weak tremors in the limbs;
- blurred vision, floaters (seeing dark specks in the field of vision); and
- scanty or delayed menses.

In Chinese medicine, the above conditions would be termed “Blood deficiency”, “Heart blood deficiency”, or “Liver blood deficiency” respectively.

In contemporary medicine, this condition would usually be called anaemia.

Dietary assistance

The following foods are all able to nourish the blood, and selected items could be added to a patient’s general diet:

- beetroot, dark leafy greens, spinach;
- date, fig, grape, apricot;
- liver, beef;
- kidney bean, aduki bean;
- chicken egg; and
- sardine, octopus, oyster.

Stomach conditions

The *Nei Jing* authors noticed that when the stomach function was weak, any of the following signs and symptoms could occur:

- nausea, vomiting, belching;
- sour regurgitation (acid reflux), hiccup;
- feeling discomfort or heat or coldness in the *epigastrium* (heartburn);

- discomfort over the ribs on the front, left side of the body (beneath which the stomach is situated), usually called indigestion;
- bleeding gums or mouth ulcers;
- bad breath—either an unpleasant odour or a burnt odour; and
- pain or discomfort anywhere along the stomach meridian.

With all the above signs and symptoms, the treatment would be very similar, and would involve the use of acupoints that strengthen the stomach function. Some key acupoints are

- Stomach-36 (on the shin, about three inches below the knee),
- Ren-12 (on the abdomen, about four inches above the navel), and
- Bladder-21 (on the back).

When poor stomach function has been present for some time, these acupoints tend to feel tender when pressed, and stimulating such acupoints encourages the stomach to cancel out the malfunction in itself that caused the tenderness.

The causes of stomach problems

Such problems often happen when a person has low energy in general, which is often due to them developing poor pancreas function; or occurs after a long illness. And once this situation is reached, the person's eating habits would then play a big part. Any of the following habits may lead to a weakening of the stomach function and the occurrence of the above signs and symptoms:

- eating too quickly and not chewing the food sufficiently;

- eating too much at one sitting, or not eating enough in general, such as when dieting;
- eating foods that are hard to digest, such as any cold or raw foods, or foods from the list on page 19; and
- being emotionally upset when eating.

Avoiding such habits would help the patient to avoid developing stomach problems. But more importantly, any weaknesses that make the patient prone to stomach problems should also be addressed, such as poor pancreas function.

Finally, as with all the organs, the stomach function can also be impeded due to mental and emotional factors. Any sustained situation in our life that we find hard to *stomach* could have this effect. In other words, when we are unable to *start* to mentally digest a fact or situation, this failure is duplicated in the stomach and impedes *its* ability to begin the process of digesting food.

Patient example
Male, aged 14. The patient's parents split up when he was aged ten, and a year later he developed stomach cramps. His elder brother then left home to attend university, which he also found hard to accept. This case was a clear example of the disruption of an organ's function due to emotional factors. He found it hard to stomach these circumstances, which then impeded his stomach function. See the full case history on page 136.

The knowledge of this particular cause-and-effect has become so clear to people over the centuries that it is now fossilized in the very language. There is no doubt that this is the origin of such expressions as: finding something *hard to stomach*, or *having no stomach* for something, or: something that *makes you sick*, where such emotions or ideas produce physical symptoms in the stomach, such as pain, nausea or indigestion.

Chapter 3. Liver and gallbladder

The liver plays a major role in the regulation, production and circulation of the resources that all our energy is created from. Consequently, when the liver ceases to function normally, this tends to produce powerful physical symptoms.

The *Nei Jing* authors noticed that when the liver function stagnates, this causes the patient to experience signs and symptoms from the following list. Not all these would be present at once, but most patients would experience a good selection of them.

- discomfort at the front or back of the torso at the level of the liver (the *hypochondrium*), frequent sighing or hiccups;
- feeling of irritability, with outbursts of angry shouting;
- muscular spasms, cramps, twitching, stiff neck;
- a feeling as though something were stuck in your throat;
- fluctuations of mood, melancholy or depression, paranoia;
- migraines or headaches with pain on the top or sides of the head or associated with the eyes, visual disturbances;
- dizziness, vertigo, hearing high pitch ringing sounds (tinnitus), insomnia;

- strong pain, stiffness or discomfort anywhere along the liver or gallbladder meridian, particularly on the head, neck, hips, outside of the legs;
- (in women) irregular periods with cramps, tender breasts, either scanty or absent menses or, alternatively, heavy flow with clots, and emotional fluctuations and irritability in the pre-menstrual phase (PMS); and (in all patients)
- effects on other organs, producing constipation, or the alternation of constipation with loose stools and other digestive signs.

Causes of stagnated liver function

Stagnated liver function (called "Liver chi stagnation" in Chinese medicine) is extremely common in developed countries, since the condition is primarily caused by mental and emotional stresses of the kind that are rife in such societies.

Chinese medicine has always recognised the connection between our thoughts and organ functions. In the body, the liver's main role is a regulatory one; and when this function is used to process our thoughts, this produces our tendency to organize the world around us. But problems result when the world declines to obey our "rules". That is, when people do not do things the way we would like, or break etiquette rules, or things are not organized as we would like. This blocks the flow of our liver-related thoughts, which the liver feels as though the physical substances in the body had stopped flowing as they should. The liver produces a powerful reaction to try to correct this blocked flow, and this is the feeling of irritation or anger that we feel when our "rules" are broken. However, our usual tendency is to suppress our anger. We may perhaps sigh, but do little else. But since the situation in our life is not resolved, the liver continues to behave as though the flow of substances and energy in our own body were also still blocked. And it is this that produces the many powerful symptoms in us (see *Acupuncture Today and in Ancient China* for more detail).

> **Patient example**
> Female, aged 32. This patient sought treatment for issues related to her menstrual cycle, primarily acne but also PMS and painful periods. All these issues were addressed by the treatment, which focused on alleviating her stagnated liver function. See the full case history on page 139.

Traits of a liver-dominated person

When our liver function is habitually stagnated, our mental activity would tend to be dominated by the "concerns" of our liver, causing the following traits to become excessive.

We would tend to *over* regulate our environment. At the simplest level, we may find ourselves frequently (almost unconsciously) adjusting the position of objects: straightening a picture on the wall or an object on our desk. And we would also tend to minutely organize every other aspect of our life. We may spend much time planning—writing lists, organizing our own and other's schedules and itineraries, organizing things such as filing systems or inventing other such systems to minutely organize the activities of everyday life, both our own and other people's.

For a person who is dominated by their liver's concerns, a major health problem is caused in them when the people (or objects) around them decline to obey their "rules". This routinely blocks their liver function, producing the following condition.

Diagnosis and treatment

When a patient has stagnated liver function they would usually have a selection of the symptoms listed on page 25 above, which the practitioner would determine by questioning. And the diagnosis would be confirmed by examining the patient's tongue and pulses.

To the practitioner, the liver pulse would resemble the feel of a taut wire under the fingers—and is called "wiry" in Chinese medicine. Some of the other organ pulses may also have this same "wiry" quality, since the stagnation often extends to the other organs as well. And the body of the patient's tongue would often have "stagnation dots" and also red sides, to one degree or another—the more pronounced the stagnation, the more this redness would be obvious. In tongue diagnosis, the left side of the tongue relates to the liver and the right to the gallbladder.

Facial colour and tone of voice

When the stagnated function is pronounced or chronic, the patient would tend to have a green facial hue which other people can often see.

The patient example on page 138 provides a striking example of this, where a boy's problems were caused by stagnated liver function, and his family reported that his complexion was notably green when his condition was at its worst.

This is also doubtless the origin of the expression "green with envy". When a person is prone to stagnated liver function, this would tend to create within them states such as envy and paranoia. The enviable situation would be seen as the breaking of "rules" (it is unfair that the other person has this desirable advantage, rather than me; it is an injustice), and the more this "injustice" were focused on, the more the person's liver function would stagnate, heightening their green hue.

The *Nei Jing* associates the liver with a "shouting" voice. When a person is prone to stagnated liver function, they would usually have a loud voice and when in normal conversation would sound as though shouting. This is a reliable diagnostic sign, and easy to recognise.

Treatment

When stagnated liver function is present, one or more of the key acupoints related to the liver tend to feel tender when pressed. The key acupoints are

- Liver-3 (on the top of the foot),
- Gallbladder-41 (on the top of the food),
- Gallbladder-34 (on the side of the leg, below the knee),
- Pericardium-6 (on the wrist; this is the familiar acupoint used for treating travel sickness),
- Liver-14 (on the chest, below the breast),
- Bladder-18 (on the back), and
- Bladder-14 (on the back).

These acupoints become tender due to their association with this particular liver malfunction. When one of these acupoints is stimulated, this encourages the organ to cancel out the malfunction in itself that caused the tenderness at the acupoint, and the organ returns to normal function.

The effect is often instant, or could sometimes takes a few minutes, when the "wiry" quality in the patient's pulses would clear, indicating the organ function was now modified. I have also noticed that any red areas on the patient's tongue also tend to clear within seconds of the liver acupoints being needled. And, of course, patient's often feel considerably less stressed at the end of the treatment, since their liver function is now more normal.

The progress of treatment

As when treating all conditions, after the first treatment the positive effects of the treatment may wear off after a day or two. But with each successive treatment, the positive effects tend to last longer. This phenomenon is partly due to resistive factors in the patient's lifestyle.

Acupuncture can "get under the radar" to address mental and emotional issues

Each person may have adopted patterns in their thinking and emotional behaviour that tend to encourage their main organs to malfunction. This is particularly so with the liver (as summarized on page 26 above), but it is also true with the other four main organs.

Their habits might include being too controlling of other people (and themselves), resulting in constant obstructed thoughts, irritability and (almost inevitably) stagnated liver function. And any difficulties might be compounded by a tendency to *not* express their frustrations or anger.

With all these patterns, there may be particular key incidents in a person's life which marked the start of the pattern, such as traumatic events; and the memory of these experiences can make it harder for the person to break the pattern. Ordinarily, mental and emotional patterns of these types would need to be changed in order for the patient's organs to return to functioning normally, and for their symptoms to thus clear—since, if these mental and emotional patterns remain the same, after every acupuncture treatment, the organs would soon re-adopt the same malfunction.

The process of us gradually changing such habits is normally a long and slow one, and with some people it may be beyond them. But acupuncture seems to "get under the radar" of our conscious mind and directly regulates the function of our main organs, which in turn tends to encourage us to spontaneously change our mental and emotional habits. I often find patients return after a few treatments and tell me about such changes; they find themselves suddenly becoming more assertive (when it is appropriate), or expressing their frustrations appropriately, or being more relaxed about which "rules" they like to see obeyed; and, in general, being more able to spot what elements in their life are bad or good for them.

However, it is still possible for a particularly strong-willed patient, who may be stuck in a mode of thinking or feeling, to doggedly cling to their familiar mental and emotional habits and thus reverse the treatments. In this situation, the patient's mind would have, in effect, blocked the treatment. With such patients, their journey in life towards good health would tend to be an extended one.

Patient example
Female, aged 28. This patient sought treatment for a neck pain. Initially her symptoms improved, but the pain returned. She continued with treatment, which gave her the clarity and courage to resolve a relationship problem, and her neck pain was then able to clear. See the full case history on page 131.

Changes to lifestyle

When receiving acupuncture treatment, patients also often spontaneously change their physical lifestyle—since the treatments seem to make them more aware of which of their habits are unhealthy. But as a general rule, long periods of inactivity are detrimental to the liver, since this encourages physical stagnation in the body, which the liver abhors. And long periods sat at a desk under stressful conditions would be particularly damaging, since the mental and emotional stresses tend to worsen the stagnation. The body is designed to be used, to be physically active during daylight hours, so incorporating a variety of physical activities into our day is key to maintaining the health of the liver—and is a great way to dissipate the effects of mental and emotional stresses. However, routine *excessive* exercise would tend to have a depleting effect on the body's key resources and in the long term could be just as damaging to our health. One of the key principles advocated by Chinese medicine is balance, in every area and aspect of life.

Other liver conditions

The following terms are also used in Chinese medicine in relation to liver conditions. Once stagnated liver function is present, this tends to affect the function of the other organs and hence the production of the blood. And once this situation has been present for some time, this may lead to signs and symptoms such as

- blurred vision, night blindness, dryness of the eyes, seeing either light specks or dark patches in the field of vision;
- poor quality nails, including soft, thin, withered, or deformed nails;
- numbness of the limbs, weak muscles;
- pale complexion, pale lips; and
- increased tendency to experience muscular cramps and spasms.

These signs and symptoms are thought to be produced by a combination of the stagnated liver function and the effects of poor quality blood, which itself came about due to the long-term stagnated liver function. In Chinese medicine, the condition is known as "Liver blood deficiency".

If the stagnated liver function eventually affects the function of the stomach, this may produce

- a feeling of indigestion (discomfort around the lower, front ribs on the left side—the location of the stomach);
- belching, nausea or vomiting, acid regurgitation; and
- a rising sensation of heat in the centre of the chest (heartburn).

In Chinese medicine, this condition is known as "Liver invading stomach".

Patient example
Male, aged 14. The patient's parents split up when he was ten, and a year later he developed stomach cramps. His elder brother then left home, which he also found hard to accept. This case provides a textbook example of "Liver invading stomach". See the full case history on page 136.

Patient example
Female, aged 32. This patient sought treatment for issues related to her menstrual cycle, primarily acne. This case also included a clear example of "Liver invading stomach", which in this case produced *heat* in the stomach which manifested itself as acne. See the full case history on page 139.

And if the function of the pancreas were affected, this could produce

- a bloated and tender abdomen,
- loose stools alternating with constipation, and
- intestinal noises.

In Chinese medicine, this condition is known as "Liver invading pancreas".

As stated on page 25 above, once the liver function has been stagnant for some time, this is likely to produce such symptoms as: constant feelings of dissatisfaction, frustration, resentment, repressed anger, possibly leading to depression. And over time, the following symptoms could also occur:

- frequent bouts of angry shouting,
- violent rages,
- migraines and headaches with severe pain, and
- dizziness, vertigo, tinnitus.

In Chinese medicine terms, this condition is known as "Liver yang rising".

Treatment of these conditions

All the above syndromes simply describe conditions that are either complications of stagnated liver function (and can therefore be successfully treated by treating that condition) or are due to problems with one of the other main organs and would be addressed by treating that organ (as well as treating the stagnated liver function), so that in the above examples, the stomach and pancreas could also be treated, as described on pages 15 and 21.

Gallbladder conditions

In contemporary physiology, the gallbladder is attached to the back of the liver by connective tissue and has the following functions.

- It acts as a reservoir for bile, which is excreted by the liver and stored in the gallbladder, ready for use in digestion.
- It concentrates the bile by extracting water from it.
- When fats are present in the duodenum (the tube through which food exits the stomach), it releases bile into the duodenum to break down the fats to aid in their digestion.

In the *Nei Jing*, the gallbladder's main function was considered to be mental—that of making decisions (see below).

Improper function

Due to the close functional link between the liver and gallbladder (bile is produced by the liver), in an acupuncture clinic it would often be impossible to determine whether certain signs and symptoms were due to malfunction of the liver or gallbladder. For example, the following signs and symptoms could be due to malfunction of either: pain in the liver region, jaundice, nausea, and a bitter taste in the mouth. However—also due to this close functional link—treating the liver with acupuncture would also treat the gallbladder, and for this reason there is not usually the need to separately consider conditions of the gallbladder.

Also due to this close relationship, acupoints on the gallbladder meridian are often used to treat liver conditions. For example, the acupoints Gallbladder-34 and Gallbladder-41 are often used to treat stagnated liver function, since (also due to this close relationship) these acupoints often become tender when the liver function stagnates.

The mental functions of the gallbladder

Through observations of mental and emotional symptoms and responses to treatment, the *Nei Jing* authors were able to observe that the gallbladder was responsible for the ability to make decisions, and the courage to act on them.

When the gallbladder is not functioning well, patients are usually indecisive and timid, which symptoms tend to clear once the gallbladder function has returned to normal. This mental function can be graphically observed in contemporary patients whose gallbladder has been surgically removed. The ones I have questioned, state that they are now unable to make the simplest of decisions, which they clearly associate with the removal of their gallbladder. Unfortunately this condition cannot be treated with acupuncture, since the treatment relies on the presence of the organ.

I have also noticed that in patients whose job involves much decision making, the gallbladder meridian on their legs is often tender when pressed; and when I test this and the patient finds it particularly tender they will often say they had a hard week at work and feel "decision fatigued". This is also noticeable in a patient who comes for treatment after having made some hard decisions recently.

Chapter 4. Lungs and large intestine

The lungs take in air directly from outside and are therefore particularly vulnerable to attack by harmful factors from outside the body. This situation produces the commonest lung condition.

Invasion by airborne pathogens

The *Nei Jing* authors noticed that when a person was exposed to airborne pathogens such as *wind* and *cold*, and their body was unable to resist the pathogens, their lung function became impaired and the person could suffer any of the following symptoms:

A. sneezing, cough, build up of mucous, nasal obstruction, watery nasal discharge, possible fever and chills, aching body, an aversion to wind and drafts, and headache.

And in some instances, the following signs and symptoms could also occur:

B. thirst, yellow mucous, sore throat, sweating, rapid pulse, and a red tongue with a thin yellow coat.

In contemporary physiology this condition is known as a cold or influenza, which is considered to be a viral infection. In Chinese medicine the condition is known as a "wind invasion", together with a description of the signs and symptoms as "cold" or "hot". If the symptoms are largely those from list "A" above, this is known as a "Wind cold invasion", but if they include some signs or symptoms from list "B", the overall condition is termed a "Wind heat invasion".

Treatment

When the lung function is impaired in this way the key lung-related acupoints tend to become tender, such as Lung-1 (below the collar bone) or Bladder-13 (on the back). Stimulating one of these acupoints encourages the lungs to cancel out the malfunction in themselves that caused these acupoints to become tender.

If the patient has a sore throat, the acupoints Lung-5 (on the inside of the elbow) or Lung-10 (near the thumb) would also tend to be tender and would be needled—for the same reason. And other features of the body's reaction to the condition would cause other acupoints to become tender, such as Bladder-12 (at the top of the back) and Large-intestine-4 (near the thumb), which are acupoints commonly used to treat a cold.

If the treatment is performed in the early stages of the cold, this can often prevent the cold developing any further and the patient returns to feeling well immediately after the treatment. I have often found that in the early stages of a cold, a hot bath, which is hot enough to induce sweating, can prevent the cold developing. At other times, I have found that simply needling the left Large-intestine-4 acupoint on myself, can have the same effect.

However, if the cold is not treated until about two or three days after the initial sneezing began, and the main symptoms are now fully developed, the treatment can only usually make the person feel more comfortable and speed up their recovery.

Retention of phlegm in the lungs

This condition tends to occur after suffering repeated attacks of colds or flu without properly recovering from each attack.

A simple cold can affect the body heavily. In a healthy person with a strong constitution, they are able to recover quickly, but many people will ignore a cold and simply continue with their normal stressful lives, not allowing themselves the opportunity to properly recover. When this pattern is repeated for years, all the main organs are likely to be affected. Such a person may develop poor functioning of the pancreas, lungs, kidneys (from constantly drawing on adrenaline to support their stressful lifestyle), and also stagnated liver function (due to the prolonged stress). With all the main organs affected, phlegm builds up in the lungs, which are unable to shift it.

In contemporary medicine, this condition would tend to be called either chronic bronchitis or bronchial asthma.

The signs and symptoms could include any combination of the following:

- recurring or persistent cough with lots of white or frothy sputum, or a cough that is loud, barking and painful, with yellow mucus which may be blood stained and strong smelling;
- shortness of breath, rattle in the throat; and
- fullness or stuffiness in the chest, sometimes with loss of appetite, nausea and vomiting, and finding it uncomfortable to lie down.

Treatment

The treatment would focus on returning the affected organs to their normal function, including the lungs, pancreas, kidneys and liver. The key acupoints to do this would have become tender, and needling them encourages the respective organs to resume their normal function. This then enables the lungs to clear the phlegm, and the digestive organs to function properly, which aids the patient's recovery. However, with any condition that is the result of chronic deficiencies (weaknesses in the function of the main organs), the condition may be slow to respond to treatment, which means that "strengthening" treatments could be required for several weeks, along with advice to the patient on changes in their lifestyle which would enable them to recover more quickly.

Poor lung function

The *Nei Jing* authors noticed that when a person had poor lung function (called "Lung chi deficiency" in Chinese medicine), they could suffer any of the following signs and symptoms:

- shortness of breath which is worse on exertion;
- weak cough with clear, thin sputum;
- poor energy and pale complexion, with an even greater energy lag between three and five p.m.;
- lack of desire to talk, having a quiet voice, and tiring quickly when having to talk a lot;
- spontaneous daytime sweating;
- frequently suffering colds and flu, and generally being easily affected by external pathogens;
- tending to feel the cold and having a dislike of being in the wind or cold;
- a poor sense of smell, blocked nose and sinuses; and
- pain or discomfort anywhere along the lung or large intestine meridian.

Face colour and tone of voice

When a person has a pronounced or chronic lung condition, their complexion would tend to be whitish. And when a person is prone to poor lung function, their voice can have a "weeping" quality, as though they were constantly sad, or about to cry.

The causes of poor lung function

This condition would tend to be present whenever the lungs are affected by an illness; or it could develop when our constitution is weakened through years of working excessively while failing to maintain an appropriate balance in life.

> **Patient example**
> Male, aged 56. This patient had poor energy due to the poor function of both his pancreas and lungs, which developed after years of driving himself too hard, which also produced poor kidney function. See the full case history on page 128.

The condition may also be present due to constitutional factors. In people who are "lung-dominant", the lung function tends to become poor due to mental factors.

The physical function of the lungs is to extract something precious (oxygen) from the air around us, and when this function is used to process our thoughts, this enables us to discern quality in the intangible things around us. People who tend to overuse this faculty, become perfectionists, but the more we look for perfection, the less we are able to find it, which creates a constant feeling of disappointment, and also weakens the lung function. When this lung function is used to process our thoughts, and it is frustrated (by not being able to extract something precious from the intangible things around us), this failure is also duplicated in the physical lung function, which makes it harder for the lungs to extract oxygen from the air around us. Hence, this constant disappointment weakens the lung function (see *Acupuncture Today and in Ancient China* for more detail).

> **Patient example**
> Male, aged 57. This patient was a perfectionist and drove himself hard in the running of his business. Over many years this caused him to develop a wide range of health issues, eventually affecting all his main organs. See the full case history on page 135.

The lungs are also weakened due to grief or any prolonged sadness, in which case poor lung function would be present. Grief is not only felt due to the loss of a loved one, but can also be felt due to the loss of anything the person cherishes, such as their job, career, social status, material possessions or wealth, and so on. When such a loss occurs, it is important that the lungs are treated to enable the person to recover from the loss; that is, to let go of the thing they cherished and move on. When a person has poor lung function, they would find it particularly difficult to go through this normal grieving process and would tend to hold on to the memory of whatever it is they had lost.

> **Patient example**
> Female, aged 65. This patient's lung function was already weak when she suffered a series of losses; first a close friend died, then her career ended, then her son died, which all affected her lung function. See the full case history on page 143.

Another factor that can lead to poor lung function is overuse of your voice. In Chinese medicine, it is recognised that one function of the lungs is to support the voice. When the lung function is weakened by illness, this can often result in the voice failing. Conversely, overuse of the voice tends to weaken the lung function.

In my practice I have treated many teachers and almost all of them had health issues related to poor lung function. Teachers not only must use their voice excessively, and often project it over a resistant and vocal class of children, but also the defensive aspect of their lungs is continuously taxed due to the prevalence of colds amongst children, and also the fact that teachers can sometimes feel "under attack" by their students—which has the same effect on us that physical pathogens do and would certainly also tax the immunity. Their lungs would also be taxed due to them having to constantly assess the quality of their students' work (teachers, by definition, are perfectionists), which also tends to weaken the lungs.

Another symptom that reflects the prevalence of lung issues amongst teachers is the fact that many teachers tend to suffer an energy lag around three p.m. This is the time of day when the lung function is at its weakest, hence the energy lag felt by people with poor lung function. This energy lag, along with any other signs and symptoms related to poor lung function, tends to clear after a few treatments (which I mention to demonstrate that this energy lag is not merely due to the fact that three p.m. is near the end of most teachers' working day).

Patient example

Male, aged 24. This patient sought treatment for migraines. He was a newly qualified teacher. He had a poor constitution due to inheriting poor kidney function from his parents, and he also had poor lung function, which caused him to experience an afternoon energy lag while at school. See the full case history on page 134.

Helpful lifestyle changes

With people whose poor lung function is not due to them overusing their voice, and are constitutionally quiet and reluctant to speak, one very effective way to improve their lung function is by using their voice more. Singing or playing a wind instrument are particularly effective.

Treating the mental factors

When there is a mental factor to the patient's condition, these usually also respond well. When a person's lung function is poor, the lung's mental functions would also be impeded and the person may find it harder to recognise quality, which may only drive them to seek it more. And any further failure to find it would weaken their lung function further, which would only fuel their obsession and lock them into a self-destructive cycle.

The lungs also actively expel the waste product of respiration (carbon dioxide), and when the lung function is used to process our thoughts, this ability enables us to let go of "waste". That is, anything in our life that may have become harmful to us. This is often something we once cherished but has now become harmful, such as relationships that have gone bad, projects we started that are not now working. But when a person's lung function is poor, this also weakens their ability to let go of this "waste" in their life. Another facet of this function is that they may bear grudges long after other people would have forgotten about the issue and moved on.

When a person is trapped in such a pattern of mental activity, it can be extremely difficult to break the pattern. But one of the strengths of acupuncture is that it prompts the physical organs to return to normal function and does this without involving our conscious mind. In effect, acupuncture seems to "get under the radar" of our conscious mind. And once the organ functions are normalized, this tends to also normalize each organ's mental functions; and after a few treatments patients often describe the changes they have spontaneously adopted in their mental behaviour.

Treatment

Due to the association between the lungs and the following acupoints, these tend to become tender when the lung function is poor. When one of these acupoints is stimulated, this encourages the organ to cancel out the malfunction in itself that caused the tenderness at the acupoint, and the organ returns to normal function:

- Lung-1 (below the collar bone),
- Bladder-13 (on the back, between the shoulder blades), and
- Bladder-42 (on the back). When the lungs are weakened by mental or emotional factors, such as grief or loss, this acupoint is often tender.

Asthma

Asthma is the contemporary term usually used to refer to all instances of breathing difficulties, but in Chinese medicine it is recognised that the underlying cause may lie in the function of either the lungs or kidneys. When the patient finds it hard to breathe out, this is usually due to poor lung function and would be treated as above. But when the patient finds it hard to breathe in, this is usually due to poor kidney function. In this case the kidneys would be treated (p.61), and treating the lungs would have no effect on the underlying cause of the condition.

Large intestine conditions

In contemporary physiology, the large intestine receives the processed food and liquid from the small intestine, moves this downward while absorbing water from it, then expels the remainder (the waste) from the body.

The most common problems related to the large intestine are either constipation or diarrhoea. These may occur for a number of reasons, most of which are due to problems in the function of other organs. For example, poor pancreas function often causes loose stools and sometimes diarrhoea (p.14); stagnated liver function can cause constipation (p.25); and general signs of *heat* in the body would also tend to dry the body fluids and lead to constipation. In all these situations, the organs involved would be treated (the pancreas, or any other organ affected), which then tends to solve the problem. But at the same time, acupoints related directly to the large intestine are also often needled, such as any of the following:

- Bladder-25 (on the lower back),
- Stomach-25 (on the abdomen, beside the navel), and
- Pancreas-15* (near to the above acupoint).

Problems due to mental factors

As with all the abdominal organs, the large intestine has mental functions, and there is a correlation between the mental functions of the large intestine and lungs. In contemporary physiology, the physical functions of both organs have similarities. The lungs sort out the precious oxygen from the air we breathe in, and the large intestine sorts out the water that it extracts from the waste of the digestion. The lungs then let go of the waste products of respiration (the carbon dioxide) and the large intestine lets go of the waste produces of digestion (the matter excreted). And because of this similarity of function, the large intestine is often *also* affected, as well as the lungs, when the mental function of "letting go of the waste" is impeded. Hence, when a person cannot mentally let go of the waste (and bears grudges for a long time, cannot let go of doomed projects or relationships, and so on), this failure of function is duplicated in the large intestine and the person becomes constipated.

As ever with acupuncture, by treating the organ, this would often enable the person to unconsciously make the necessary changes in their mental patterns, and once they were able to mentally "sort the good from the bad" and "let go of the waste", their large intestine function would also tend to return to normal.

---

* Also called Spleen-15.

Damage due to improper food intake

It was noticed that when a person ate excessive amounts of raw and cold foods, or "unclean" foods (dirty water or rotten foods), this could produce any combination of the following signs and symptoms:

- abdominal pain;
- stools that have a foul smell with blood or mucus, *or* diarrhoea with yellow, watery stools (the diarrhoea starts suddenly and urgently, and the desire may continue afterwards, even though the bowels are empty);
- burning sensation in the anus; and
- there may also be thirst, fever, dark urine, and a rapid pulse and red tongue with a yellow coating.

In Chinese medicine terms, the condition is known as "Damp heat invading the large intestine". In contemporary medicine, this same condition would probably be called bacillary dysentery.

Treatment

The acupoints mentioned above (Bladder-25, Stomach-25 and Pancreas-15) may be used to treat any condition affecting the large intestine, including this one, but in particular, the following acupoint would usually also be added:

- Stomach-37 (below the knee). This acupoint has been found to treat a wide range of conditions affecting the large intestine, and in particular to alleviate diarrhoea and dysenteric disorder.

Chapter 5. Kidneys and bladder

When the "kidneys" are mentioned in Chinese medicine, this is referring to three structures that are today regarded as separate organs: the kidneys, adrenal glands and gonads.

The adrenal glands are attached to the top of the kidneys, and the gonads are nearby. These three organs all share the same meridian, which is known as the kidney meridian, so that when kidney acupoints are stimulated, this is able to treat all three of these structures. From the physiological point of view, these three structures may all therefore be considered to be the same, single organ.

In contemporary physiology, the main functions of the kidneys are to

- filter out various toxins from the blood;
- regulate the amount of water that circulates in the blood plasma;
- recycle other vital nutrients in the body, such as glucose and amino acids;
- help to martial the body's resources in times of stress, by constricting the blood vessels to increase blood pressure;
- regulate the amount of red blood cells; and to
- work closely with the lungs to regulate the acid level (pH) in the body.

The adrenal glands function differently depending on whether the body is stressed or not.

When not stressed, their main functions are to

- regulate the body's energy usage and mobilize its energy stores;
- regulate the blood glucose level, by counteracting insulin;
- play a key role in the development and maintenance of normal immunity; and to
- enable the brain to create short term memories.

And when the body is stressed, the main functions of the adrenal glands are to

- suppress the immune system and bone formation, slow down the healing of wounds, and shut down the reproductive system;
- actively increase the immediate supply of energy; and to
- raise blood pressure levels.

The gonads are the testes (in men) and the ovaries (in women). Between them they secrete hormones that control the body's development at each stage of life—as we pass from childhood into puberty and on into adulthood and old age.

The thoughts produced by the kidney function

In contemporary physiology the "kidneys" (considering all three kidney-related structures as a whole) are mainly concerned with our self-preservation, both in the present and the future. Amongst other functions, the kidneys coordinate our growth and development, from conception through to adulthood; are the key reproductive organ, being responsible for fertility and our sexual behaviour, which thus provides us with our engagement in life, the desire to go on living and the tendency to form goals and have the determination to see them through. They regulate the body's energy usage, so as to ensure the proper function of all the organs, thus enabling us to function at our best in the present and also enabling us to deal with stressful situations; and they manage and support the immunity.

Considering all these factors, the kidneys' physical function could be summarized as: *to* (produce the desire to) *want to be alive and continue living; to reproduce, set goals for the future and pursue those goals; and to recognise threats and find a solution to them* (which is the role played by the immunity). This wording also serves as a summary of the kidneys' logic; and when this logic is used to process our thoughts, what thought patterns might result?

Our motivation in many areas of life

The kidney function to *reproduce, set goals for the future and pursue those goals* produces every aspect of our sexual behaviour, all our actions and thoughts concerning our attraction to others and making ourselves attractive to *them*. This could cause us to modify our appearance or seek such things as status or certain achievements, all of which we may consider—even if only subconsciously—could enhance our attractiveness. And when the kidney function drives us *to set goals for the future and to pursue them*, we may often feel the desire to be doing or producing something that we feel is "worthwhile", or wanting to achieve something that makes us feel good about ourselves. Both these are very similar motivations to that of wanting to improve our status or attractiveness. But at other times, our only motivation may be seeking to enjoy the simple pleasure of being alive, which is produced in us by the kidney function *to want to be alive and continue living*. And another common motivation is the desire to leave something behind, which is produced by this same function: the kidneys' desire for us to go on living.

The kidney function *to recognise threats and find a solution to them* was originally evolved to protect us from predators. This still applies today, on the occasions when we might be faced with an actual predator (such as an aggressive animal or person), but this also applies to other threats, such as illnesses (causing us to avoid an ill person) or dangerous situations. And this also applies whenever any aspect of our status, or the safety of anything or anyone we care about is threatened. In any of these situations, this kidney function produces our feeling of fear and also focuses our resources (by releasing adrenaline) to enable us to tackle the threat.

The kidneys produce fear

Through practical observations, the *Nei Jing* authors noticed that the emotion of fear was produced by the kidneys.

Just as whenever the *liver* function is obstructed and the liver produces the emotion of anger to attempt to remove the obstruction; so, when the kidney function is undermined (perhaps some element of our safety or status, or a cherished person or thing, is threatened), the kidneys produce the emotion of fear to cause us to take urgent action to remedy the situation. This might be to flee from the danger or take evasive action to remove the threat. Fear is produced in two main situations.

1. When the kidney function becomes weak

When the kidney function is poor, this makes us less resilient, reduces our stamina, weakens the function of *all* the organs, as well as reducing the availability of energy generally. All these things are regulated by the "kidneys"; hence any weakness in the kidney function could produce these effects. This places us in a vulnerable state. One of the kidney functions is *to want to be alive and continue living*, and when we feel vulnerable, this undermines this function, so the kidneys produce the emotion of fear to prompt us to address the situation.

This would start as a state of general fearfulness, rather than a sudden fright, but it would also be accompanied by a release of adrenaline. This state can be frequently seen in people. When they become drained (often through driving themselves too hard), they tend to become jumpy, and their sensitivity to sounds may also become more acute—hearing is the sense the kidneys are most closely associated with.

This is a defensive state; we are made more alert, so we can watch out for danger and are able to respond quickly to it, should we spot it. Ordinarily, this is intended only as a short-term measure, but when this state becomes almost constant, it only weakens the kidneys further—through overuse of these emergency reserves. This then only increases our fearfulness, increases our general depletion and inhibits the good function of all the organs, all of which diminishes our long-term health.

The stage of life when poor kidney function is common is old age, which is why old people are often fearful—which constant state of fearfulness only tends to weaken their kidney function even further. If longevity is a concern of yours, then avoiding fearful situations at *all* stages in life would be beneficial.

2. When we notice a threat

Another of the kidney functions is *to reproduce, set goals for the future and pursue those goals.* This also goes hand in hand with its function *to want to be alive and continue living.*

When we notice anything that threatens our own physical safety, or that of our loved ones, or threatens our social position or our achievements, this undermines these kidney functions. In response, the kidneys produce the emotion of fear to prompt us to address the threat—and the degree of fear would reflect the urgency of the threat.

In contemporary physiology, the adrenal glands are heavily associated with the "flight" response, and since the adrenal glands are one of the three kidney-related structures, this also supports the associations between fear, flight, self preservation and the kidneys.

The kidney function is also used to *process* the threatening situation. One part of its function is to *recognise threats and find a solution to them.* This kidney logic (in other words, the "logic" of the immune system) is then used to quickly process the situation and present a solution to our conscious mind.

The "immune system" can also process our thoughts

Supposing the threat were to our physical safety, the solution might be the idea that we should flee the danger, should move aside and dodge it. Or, if the threat was from another person or an animal that we could combat, the solution may be to fight it. Or the threat may be a comment a person made which appeared to put us in jeopardy in some way. This may be by threatening our position, our notions of our own status or worth, or the security of our job or our relationships or something else we cared deeply about. In this situation, the kidneys' solution may be to work out a lie for us to tell to fend off the danger, and this lie would then pop into our mind. It is common to see people reacting in this way, when they will clearly enter an adrenaline-fuelled state and spontaneously lie to protect themselves from any perceived threat.

In other situations, people may respond to a threat by working out a course of action to discredit the person who appears to be attacking them. If this course of action occurs to them spontaneously, within a second or so of them perceiving the threat, it would have most likely been worked out by the immune-system aspect of their kidney function. But sometimes, people can dwell on such threats for hours or days, until the solution eventually pops into their mind. In this situation, the solution would have usually been worked out by their liver function, using the liver's creative ability—to remove this "obstruction to the flow of their thoughts".

Another way the kidney function may be utilized mentally is in spotting opportunities to further its goals. These might be in the workplace or socially. Suppose you were in a work situation and your superior said something, and in response an idea popped into your head about something you could say or do that would advance your position, either in the eyes of your boss or your company generally. This idea, which appeared to spontaneous occur to you, was produced by your kidney function. The same situation may occur to us socially. Your partner, or an admired friend, may say or do something, and in response an idea may spontaneously pop into your head about something you could say or do to curry favour with them. Again, this idea would have been produced by the logic of your kidneys.

This type of spontaneous idea is often accompanied by a release of adrenaline, which reinforces the notion that the idea originates in the "kidneys".

We have all experienced this phenomenon, but as to whether or not we act on the idea is another matter—some people do and some do not. Another common example is when we see an object unattended, which we regard as having value. It might be money, or a phone or laptop computer or item of jewellery or simply an object that only we cherish and which is of little value to anyone else, such as an object of no intrinsic value but which we consider collectable. In this situation, the idea may pop into our mind to commit an opportunistic theft—and may be accompanied by a surge of adrenaline, which may be proportionate to the value the object has in *our* eyes. Such ideas are produced by the kidney function. We have all experienced this, but, again, whether or not we act on the idea would be determined by other "voices" within us. These may be produced by the logic of the lungs, liver, or heart—which consider such matters as quality, including the quality of our own behaviour in *our* eyes; our sense of obeying the rules, of what is wrong or right; and our feelings towards other people. And it is also these same "voices" that determine whether or not we act on this type of spontaneous idea in social or work situations.

If a situation is urgent, the kidneys tend to respond—since they are mostly concerned with our self-preservation and dealing with immediate threats. Whereas if the situation is not urgent, but a niggling preoccupation, then it is the liver that tends to respond—since it is primarily concerned with keeping substances moving in the body and removing any obstructions to that flow; and here the "substances" are our ideas and thoughts.

How this affects our health

On the mental and emotional level, the role of the kidneys is to, in effect, manage the balance between fear and drive. Sometimes our drive is in response to fear. For example, we may fear losing our job if we do not work excessively hard and long hours, or we may fear losing a friendship or romantic relationship if we do not constantly work hard at it. This type of drive is unhealthy; it would be accompanied by an adrenaline release, which would assist us to perform but over time would tend to weaken the kidneys (through overuse of this emergency resource) which in turn would produce poor kidney function with a *selection* of the physical signs and symptoms listed on page 59 below.

Patient example

Male, aged 57. This patient drove himself hard. He ran his own business, and due to the responsibilities he took on single-handedly, he felt unsupported. This produced a sense of fear for his long-term survival which impeded his kidney function and also caused serious low-back problems. See the full case history on page 135.

Once a person has poor kidney function, the mental and emotional functions of the kidneys would also function poorly, causing the person to see threats in situations which other people would not consider threatening. This would only cause them to work that much harder (whether in a social or work context), which would tend to weaken their kidney function even further, causing extra or stronger physical symptoms, and possibly causing the work or social relationships to become strained. This would then only increase the perception of danger and the tendency to drive themselves too hard.

On the other hand, drive can often be healthy, provided it is not excessive. When we are driven to do a certain thing through pure excitement alone, or interest in that activity, this can be invigorating. It evokes the kidney function of *regulating and enabling the functioning of the other organs*—in other words, providing our "spark". It can make us feel energized and alive. This type of drive has no element of fear and is usually only beneficial, provided an appropriate balance is practised in every area of your life—including allowing yourself enough relaxation and an appropriate amount of physical exercise and an adequate diet. But when the drive becomes excessive (even though driven by excitement alone) this would also weaken the person's kidneys and could produce any of the signs and symptoms of poor kidney function.

When our spirit is defeated

Another common health problem related to the mental aspect of the kidneys is when our spirit is defeated. The kidney logic identifies our goals in life, our ambitions, and fosters our ideas about our worth, status, or position in life; and the kidneys then drive us to achieve these ambitions. But when any of our ambitions are defeated, or our status or position in life is taken away, this undermines these kidney functions in our thoughts, which undermining is duplicated in the kidneys, impeding their physical function.

In this situation, the person's "spark" would be clearly diminished; they would become gloomy, dispirited. The kidney function of regulating the production of energy would become poor and consequently the other main organs would function poorly. The person would become sluggish, would certainly be melancholic or in a depressive state (as though their body had been shut down) and they may feel like giving up on life, having no drive or spirit.

In such patients, the kidney acupoints on their chest would tend to be tender when pressed, and needling these can often visibly restore the patient's spirit during that session. The key acupoints are Kidney-24 and Kidney-25. Historically, in China acupoints were known by names, rather than using the numbering system we use today, and the names often indicate the use of the acupoint. Interestingly, in the case of these two acupoints, these were called "spirit ruin" and "spirit storehouse" respectively, indicating that they tended to become tender when a person's spirit was damaged, and could therefore be used to rectify the situation. That is, to normalize the aspect of the kidney function that was undermined by the mental or emotional shock.

> **Patient example**
> Male, aged 51. This patient took a break from treatment for three years. When he next came, he was like a broken man and seemed noticeably aged. He had been through a divorce and felt the financial loss greatly. The acupoint Kidney-24 was very tender when pressed. I needled this, and other acupoints, and at the end of the session he looked about five years younger and the sparkle had returned to his eyes; he said he felt like a new person.

Dietary factors

The *Nei Jing* authors noticed that salt "resonates" with the kidneys. In other words, salt nourishes the kidneys and a certain amount of salt intake is essential for the kidneys to remain healthy. Because of this, people with poor kidney function often crave salty foods. But as with all aspects of Chinese medicine, balance is the key. If too much salt were eaten this would have a depleting effect on the kidneys. However, many people in developed countries have been mislead into thinking that *all* salt is bad and should be avoided at all cost. This is equally wrong. Apart from the fact that correct seasoning enhances the taste of food and so increases the pleasure we gain from it, salt is an essential mineral for our health.

Drinking too much water can also damage the kidneys, and many people have also been mislead into thinking they must drink a large amount of water each day. In general this is also wrong and would tend to weaken the kidneys. Extra water should be drunk only when you feel thirsty.

In contemporary physiology, salt deficiency is called *hyponatremia*, and is recognised as being associated with such conditions as poor mental development in children and poor mental function and brain damage in adults (all of which the *Nei Jing* authors associated with poor kidney function), and it is also recognised that this condition can be caused in adults by drinking too much water, which again correlates with this ancient (but forgotten) knowledge.

Improper function

In Chinese medicine, the main condition that affects the kidneys is poor kidney function (also called "Kidney chi deficiency", or other terms—listed on page 63), which would tend to produce a *selection* of the following signs and symptoms:

A. Soreness and weakness of the lower back (lumbar region), and weak knees or stiff joints; frequent and urgent urination (it cannot be put off), and dribbling of urine after urination, or incontinence (enuresis); premature ejaculation in men; hay fever and other allergies, frequent colds and flu; dizziness or lightheaded feeling (particularly after sex in men); oedema, particularly in the lower half of the body; low-pitch tinnitus (or rumbling or swishing sounds); deafness or being hard of hearing; loss of balance; tendency to feel fearful; craving salty food.

B. Shortness of breath, asthma (where it is difficult to breathe in*).
C. Insomnia; poor short term memory; thirst, afternoon fever (hot flushes) and night sweating, dry mouth, hot hands and feet.
D. Cold limbs, aversion to cold; low energy and apathy.
E. Slow physical development, poor skeletal development, brittle bones, poorly formed or loose teeth; slow mental development; mental dullness, premature senility, dementia; premature greying and hair loss; impotence, infertility.

Face colour, tone of voice, and food craving

The *Nei Jing* authors associated kidney conditions with a facial colour described as resembling "violet wrapped up in white silk," which would be particularly prevalent beneath the eyes. The person would also tend to have a "groaning" tone of voice, and to crave salty food.

Causes of poor kidney function

In most people this condition develops as a normal part of the aging process. Indeed all the classic signs of old age are due to poor kidney function (deafness, loss of teeth and hair, infertility, low back ache, weak knees, brittle bones, incontinence, frequent urination, low energy or "slow movements", lack of drive, poor short term memory, senility, dementia). But the

* Difficulty in breathing *out* is due to poor lung function (p.45).

kidney function can also be weakened for the other reasons mentioned above (p.56 onwards): through driving ourselves too hard; by our spirit being defeated; or the condition can be inherited from our parents.

> **Patient example**
> Male, aged 24. This patient had a ten-year history of migraines. He inherited poor kidney function from his parents, which caused childhood hay fever and poor hearing, and also left him with a weak constitution, which made him prone to migraine attacks later in life. See the full case history on page 134.

Treatment

When the kidney function is poor, this causes various acupoints to become tender—due to their association with the kidneys. When one of these acupoints is stimulated, this encourages the organ to cancel out the malfunction in itself that caused the tenderness at the acupoint, and the organ returns to normal function. In this way, the problem is corrected by the organ itself. The key acupoints are:

- Kidney-3 (behind the ankle),
- Kidney-6 (beneath the ankle),
- Kidney-1 (on the sole of the foot),
- Ren-4 (below the navel),
- Bladder-23 (on the lower back),
- Du-4 (on the lower back), and
- Heart-7 (on the wrist).

Moxibustion

Moxibustion is a technique that is very effective when treating the kidneys. This is the application of heat to the acupoints using a stick containing powered *mugwort*, which is usually used in addition to needling those acupoints. The energy contained in the heat seems to be communicated to the associated organ, greatly increasing the strength of its function.

With "deficient" conditions, moxibustion tends to be a very effective addition to the treatment.

General prognosis

Due to the nature of poor kidney function (it being a condition where the patient's core resources have become depleted, or where they were born with inadequate core resources) recovery tends to be slower than with conditions related to the other main organs. Still, with many patients great success can be achieved after a course of about six treatments. This is even the case when the condition has developed as a part of the aging process; I have treated many elderly patients who have gained relief from many of their kidney-related symptoms. But with patients who inherited poor kidney function from their parents, it is sometimes not possible to *permanently* normalize their kidney function. In these cases, after the initial course of treatments, the patients may need to return for a maintenance treatment once a month or so if they wish to maintain good health. This would depend on each patient; the more they were able to adjust their lifestyle to match their limited physical resources, the less they would require further treatments. This often happens spontaneously anyway, since the treatments seem to make patients more aware of things in their life that are wrong for them—and they start to make appropriate changes. With *all* patients, the more they were able to do this, the less they would require follow-up treatments—though maintaining the perfect balance in life is not an easy task in developed countries, where many aspects of life can often be stressful.

Asthma

The underlying cause of asthma is often poor kidney function. This would be the case when the patient finds it hard to breathe in. When patients find it hard to breathe out, this would usually be due to poor lung function. It is important to establish which of these two types the patient has, so the condition can be effectively and quickly treated. If the kidney function is the problem, the patient would be likely to also suffer a selection of signs and symptoms from those listed on page 59 above, and the shortness of breath would often be worse between five and seven a.m., which is when the kidney function is at its weakest.

Other Chinese medicine terms used for kidney conditions

In today's Chinese medicine, poor kidney function is usually called "Kidney chi deficiency". And when certain signs and symptoms predominate, several other terms are also used. For example, most patients would tend to suffer *some* of the signs and symptoms from list "A" on page 59 above, but if they *also* suffered some from one of the other lists, then a different Chinese medicine term may be used to describe the condition instead. If symptoms from list "B" were also suffered, the term "Kidney failing to receive chi" could be used; or if symptoms from list "C", the term "Kidney yin deficiency" could be used; or if symptoms from list "D", the term "Deficient kidney yang" could be used; or if signs and symptoms from list "E", the term "Deficient kidney essence" or "Deficient kidney jing" could be used.

It should be noted that the above terms were not used in the *Nei Jing* and have been adopted more recently. They are specific to the recent practice of Chinese medicine.

However, each of the terms is simply indicating that the patient has poor kidney function with signs and symptoms in a certain area tending to predominate. And in all cases the treatment is almost identical anyway, so (in line with the general *Nei Jing* practice) this book simply lists a single kidney condition: poor kidney function.

Bladder conditions

In contemporary physiology, the function of the bladder is to temporarily store and then excrete urine, which is produced by the kidneys. The kidneys filter out various toxins from the blood, and also some of the waste products of the normal chemical activity in the body, such as urea.

The *Nei Jing* authors considered the bladder to be a storage place for body liquids. In their theories of metabolism, there was no notion that the blood needed to be filtered, nor that the kidneys performed any such function. This is understandable, since their theories were formed over 2,000 years ago, long before today's knowledge of chemistry and of the microscopic anatomy of the organs existed. Instead, their key knowledge was based entirely on practical observation, which is why much of it still remains true today, forms the core of Chinese acupuncture, and contains many important health insights, yet to be equalled by contemporary medicine.

Treating the bladder

The *Nei Jing* authors recognised that the strength of the bladder function was dependent on the strength of the kidney function. When the kidney function was poor, the patient would suffer such symptoms as frequent and urgent urination and incontinence; and after the kidney function was treated, these symptoms would clear. This symptomatic association between the two organs is so strong that, in Chinese medicine terms, such symptoms are seen as symptoms of poor kidney function, rather than of poor bladder function. And due to this symptomatic link between the two organs, the bladder is usually regarded as merely an extension of the kidneys, with no need for it to be treated, or considered, separately. However, one fairly common bladder condition requires separate mention.

Burning sensation on urination

The usual symptoms are: burning sensation on urination, with cloudy, deep yellow, strong smelling urine; and there is usually also poor kidney function, which may cause various other signs and symptoms from the list on page 59 above. The condition is usually treated with a selection of the following acupoints:

- Bladder-23 (on the lower back),
- Bladder-28 (on the sacrum),
- Ren-3 (below the navel),
- Pancreas-6* (on the lower calf), and
- Pancreas-9† (below the knee).

In my experience, the treatment is extremely effective and the main symptom (the burning sensation on urination) is often cleared with a single treatment.

In today's Chinese medicine, this condition is called "Damp heat in the bladder", which can be understood as follows.

The terms "dampness", "heat" and "damp heat"

The Chinese medicine term of *dampness* may be explained as follows. In contemporary physiology, this may be visualized as the improper regulation of the glucose, fats and proteins circulating in the blood, which then denies the organs and systems of the body proper nutrition, which, in time, may impede certain aspects of the kidney function, resulting in oedema.

In Chinese medicine, this state is regarded as pathogenic; that is, the *dampness* itself is regarded as a pathogen. Simplis-

* Also called Spleen-6.

† Also called Spleen-9.

tically, this could be visualized as the "soup" of nutrients in the blood being too thick.

The Chinese medicine term *heat* simply means any unusual warmth in the body—which could be generated by the body's reaction to a pathogen, or by the malfunction of the organs or bodily tissue. The warmth is generated by our own body and is often accompanied by redness and swelling.

When such *heat* is produced in response to *dampness*, the condition is known as *damp heat*. Regarding the symptom of "burning on urination", the *heat* would be the symptom produced in the kidneys due to their function being impeded by the *dampness* (i.e. the improper regulation of the organ's nutrition).

The acupoints I mentioned above are used to remedy the condition as follows. Pancreas-6 and Pancreas-9 strengthen the digestion, so that less *dampness* is produced, and the accumulated *dampness* clears more quickly; Bladder-23 and Bladder-28 are used to strengthen the kidney and bladder functions respectively; and Ren-3, which is directly over the bladder and is able to directly "vent" the *heat* from the bladder (though there are other explanations for how this "venting" is actually achieved).

Patient example

Female, aged 32. This patient sought treatment for issues related to her menstrual cycle, primarily acne but also PMS and painful periods; and she also had recurring thrush, with a burning sensation on urination. In this case the thrush was due to *damp heat*. See the full case history on page 139.

One of the assets of Chinese medicine is that it can treat such conditions by referring to general concepts such as *heat* and *damp heat*, without having to define the condition in microscopic terms. Instead, it simply prompts the organs to return to normal function, and the organs themselves make any chemical, hormonal, or other adjustments necessary.

In contemporary physiology, such a condition is said to be caused by a bacterial or viral "infection", which appears to suggest that such a condition ought not to respond to having an acupuncture needle inserted in the skin. However, the treatment is extremely effective and has been used for thousands of years, which highlights one of the common problems encountered when attempting to understand this ancient healing system using concepts from contemporary physiology.

On page 153, further reading is described which provides more detail of the translation of Chinese medicine concepts such as *heat* into the concepts used in contemporary physiology, and also explains (in this same context) how acupuncture successfully treats bacterial and viral infections.

Chapter 6. Heart and small intestine

In contemporary physiology, it is now known that the heart provides the force to move the blood. However, it was not until 1628 AD that William Harvey discovered this function of the heart and the existence of the blood circulatory system. Therefore, in ancient China no such concept was known to exist. The *Nei Jing* authors did not consider the heart to act as a pump, nor that the blood needed any propulsive power added to it; it was considered to propel itself, perhaps much as a river was thought to do. Instead, using their practical approach, the *Nei Jing* authors noticed that one of the heart's main functions was that it worked closely with the lungs, as follows. They noticed that when the heart function was poor, the following symptoms (amongst others) could occur:

- shortness of breath,
- profuse sweating,
- chills, and
- listlessness or lassitude.

They also noticed that when the lung function was poor, the following, similar symptoms could occur:

- shortness of breath,
- sweating,

- feeling cold, and
- lack of energy.

When stressed, either of the organs could produce these very similar symptoms. The main factor that differentiates between the two organs is that if the lungs produce the symptoms, the patient also has a cough; but if the heart produces the symptoms, the patient has palpitations. Since both organs could produce very similar symptoms, it must have seemed to the *Nei Jing* authors that the function of the two organs was inextricably linked, and this idea was expressed in their metabolic theories.

In contemporary physiology, there is also close cooperation between the heart and lungs, in the *pulmonary circulation.* The deoxygenated blood from the body returns to the heart via the *venae cavae* (the two largest veins in the body) enters the right *atrium* of the heart. It then passes to the heart's right *ventricle* and is pumped into the *pulmonary artery.* This carries the deoxygenated blood to the lungs (the pulmonary artery divides into two, to supply each lung). Within the lungs the pulmonary arteries divide into smaller arteries, *arterioles* and *capillaries.* Gas exchange then takes place between the air in the *alveoli* of the lungs, and the blood in the capillaries (oxygen passing from the air into the blood, and CO_2 passing from the blood into the air). The capillaries which contain the oxygenated blood, join up to form two veins in each lung, the *pulmonary veins,* which then leave each lung and return the oxygenated blood to the left atrium of the heart. This passes into the left ventricle and is pumped out into the *aorta,* which is the first artery of the general blood circulation in the body.

This validates the *Nei Jing* authors' observations. Having no knowledge of this close "plumbing" between the heart and lungs, they managed, over two thousand years ago, to deduce that this close cooperation existed by merely observing symptoms.

The heart's association with the tongue and faculty of speech

The *Nei Jing* authors also noticed that when a person had poor heart function, they would often also have speech defects (such as stammering or stuttering) which cleared once the heart was successfully treated, and this association is still routinely encountered in clinic today. This suggests that the good function of the heart is essential for our speech to work smoothly.

The heart's mental and emotional functions

In contemporary physiology, the main physical function of the heart is to circulate blood to every other organ and part of the body, through the system of arteries and veins. This function could be summarized in words as: *to reach out to those around it and spread nourishment to them*, where "those around it" refers to the other organs. And this wording could also be used to summarize the heart's mental function.

The thoughts produced by the heart function

In our mental and emotional lives, there are two main situations in which this function is applied. The first is when we feel concern for other people or feel affection for our friends or loved ones; and the second is when we feel the desire to share our knowledge or good fortune with others.

When we feel concern for another person, we can often sense that this emotion originates from the heart; and when sensing this, some people even physically clutch their chest over the heart region. This knowledge has clearly existed in society for a long time, since it is fossilized in the language, in phrases such as "my heart goes out to them". And whenever we care for someone in this way, we may also experience a "warm glow" in our heart. Why do we feel this sensation?

The heart function is *to reach out to other people and spread nourishment to them*, and when this function is used to process our thoughts, this produces our concern for other people. This concern is probably the strongest mental expression of the heart function we could make; and this emphasizes the heart function in our thoughts. This emphasis is then duplicated in the heart, causing us to feel that warm glow. That is, the heart feels unusually energized. This is similar to the way the heart may feel after a bout of physical exercise; that is, a bout of vigorously spreading nourishment to those around it (the other organs).

This effect happens even if we only *think* fondly of another person, so that just the idea itself is able to enhance the heart function and produce that warm glow within it.

When we simply talk to other people, a similar effect happens. Again, we are *reaching out to other people and spreading nourishment to them.* In the human context, this nourishment simply involves information about the world. In creatures who do not have the faculty of speech, the sounds they produce would constitute "nourishment" in some other way. Much of the animal sounds that have been understood by us (including bird song and the sounds produced by many mammals) are clearly providing information about the world to the other creatures around them, such as warnings of possible danger and so on.

You may have noticed that when talking to someone socially, you can sometimes feel a sensation like a mild glow within your heart—it feels good to talk. But when merely listening to the other person, this feeling is not there. It seems it is the action of *spreading information to others* that produces this effect, no matter what the information is. The act of simply talking to others appears to engage our heart function mentally, which then enhances the heart's physical function.

How this affects the health of the heart

As well as the heart function being enhanced in this way, the reverse is also possible. When the heart logic is used to process our thoughts but that logic is impeded or blocked by our conscious mind, this situation is duplicated in the heart which then behaves as though its *physical* function were being impeded. There are many situations in our daily lives where this scenario could apply.

Suppose you feel concern for someone (which may be an unfortunate person you see in the street, or a friend or work colleague who is in a difficult situation) but instead of acting on your concern and doing something to help them, you walk away. In this situation, your concern was produced by your heart's intention, which wanted to *reach out to those around you and spread nourishment to them.* And when your conscious mind overruled this emotion and you walked away, this impeded your heart's intention and hence also its physical function, which may have caused you to feel a physical pang in your heart as you walked away. That feeling was the physical discomfort your heart felt when its function was impeded. And if, after the event, you kept recalling that unfortunate person's plight, your heart would continue to feel the discomfort of having its function impeded. In this situation, you might sometimes be so aware of your heart's discomfort that this causes you to finally do something to help the person, which would then remove this impediment to your heart function and bring relief.

Suppose that during the course of your work you were required to adopt a position you knew was morally wrong. You knew that the right thing to do was to reach out and assist a person in some way but your particular work role required you to overrule your emotions and do the opposite. Or suppose you decided to be dishonest towards a particular person, or in a particular situation. In all these types of situations, your heart's intention to *reach out to those around you and spread nourishment to them*, is impeded and consequently your heart's *physical* function would be impeded. You might feel "heavy in the heart", or as though a "dark cloud" were passing over your heart. Or with some people this impediment to their heart function would immediately affect their speech (due to the association between our heart and speech) and at the instant they started lying, or saying something they felt was morally wrong, or simply adopting a position they knew was morally wrong, they might start to stutter or stammer.

This happens with people who otherwise have no problem with their heart function (what we might call "normal" people in their everyday lives) but because they adopt this conduct that they know to be morally wrong, this impedes their heart's intention (preventing it from *reaching out to those around them and spreading nourishment to them*), which impediment is duplicated in their physical heart, and since our speech is dependent on the good functioning of the heart, they develop a mild stammer or stutter, which clears when they change the topic of conversation.

The heart also uses sight to communicate

When we consciously overrule our heart's intention in this way, we might also be unable to look the other person in the eye. This action of us looking the other person in the eye is another expression of the heart's intention to *reach out to them and spread nourishment to them*; but in this case the connection is made by using eyesight as the means of communication. But since our conscious mind has impeded the heart's intention (by us being dishonest, and so on), it also impedes our ability to look the other person in the eye. The fact that the heart also uses eyesight as a means of communication is reflected in the meridian paths. There is said to be two internal meridians that ascend from the heart and one then connects with the root of the tongue while the other connects with the eyes. There would seem to be no anatomical reason why the heart should possess a meridian link to the eyes, so that this may reflect the fact that the heart also uses the eyesight to communicate.

The connection between the organ functions and our thoughts is immediate

These physical effects usually occur instantly; we feel the heaviness in our heart or the detriment to our speech or our inability to make eye contact, the moment our conscious mind chooses to overrule the heart's intention. This demonstrates just how direct the connection is between the heart's physical function and any of our thought processes that utilize the heart's logic.

These effects, though, would be felt to different degrees by different people. The more sensitive a person is, the more likely they would be to notice any impediments in their social connections, and therefore the more likely it would be for their speech to be affected by such things, or for the degree of their speech impediment to be greater.

Another example of an impediment in our connection to *those around us* is when we are involved in a dispute of any kind. Because our connection to those people is "faulty", this fault is duplicated in the heart function.

> **Patient example**
> Male, aged 49. This patient initially sought treatment following chest pains. He suffered a suspected heart attack and was found to have an inflamed pericardium. He was involved in a long-standing serious dispute with one of his neighbours, which had certainly caused a pain in the patient's jaw and probably also contributed to his heart problems. See the full case history on page 141.

Another obvious example of this phenomenon is when a relationship or friendship ends. This type of relationship is probably the most powerful mental and emotional expression of our heart's intention to *reach out to those around us and spread nourishment to them.* And we would have built a large part of our lives around that particular connection, which is then suddenly broken. Such a break is probably the greatest impediment that could be made to the mental application of the heart's intention, which impediment is duplicated in the physical heart, causing us to experience an intense pain in the heart and (with sensitive people) possibly even palpitations (see the case histories on pages 143-145, where palpitations and panic attacks were triggered by such a loss).

Loneliness weakens the heart

A similar situation is loneliness. This involves, in effect, our conscious suppressing of the heart's intention to *reach out to those around us.* This is a fundamental aspect of the heart's intention and when we mentally block it, or impede it, this impediment is duplicated in the physical heart which produces that feeling of "heaviness" in our heart—the physical pain of loneliness.

It is certainly possible to die of a "broken heart" or to eventually die from loneliness; such a death would usually occur due to a heart attack. Heart attacks have always been far more common amongst men than women. This is probably because, socially, men have always been much more alone than women. In most societies it is the normal practice for women to talk to one another about their emotional concerns, or about anything that troubles them. But with men, such talk is usually discouraged and even socially frowned upon. This creates in them a great sense of loneliness. Ultimately, they have no-one to confide in and must cope alone with whatever troubles they have. Due to social pressures, their conscious mind suppresses their heart's intention to *reach out to those around them*, and in doing this they impede their heart's physical function. Eventually this can lead to a heart attack.

It is also notable that speech defects such as stammering or stuttering are much more common amongst men than women, which seems to reflect the fact that men are required by most societies to adopt a persona that is bad for their heart.

It is possible that the circulatory system may have evolved due to the expression of the heart's intention. Its desire to *reach out to those around it and spread nourishment to them* may have resulted in the evolution of the arteries and other blood vessels—spreading out from the heart and feeding the other organs and every tissue in the body. In people who suffer heart attacks, they sometimes also have diseases of their blood vessels. Or some people may suffer serious arterial disease before any pronounced defect is noticed in their heart. In such people, their social connections with the people around them would have often been severely impeded (or "faulty") for years. These social connections are the mental expression of the heart function, and any impediment in this mental expression is duplicated in the heart, producing poor heart function, but also—since the fault is in our *connection* with other people—producing faults in the arteries and veins (which are the heart's connections to the other organs and areas of the body). In other words, our social connections are diseased, so our physical blood vessels become diseased.

Simply talking, or helping others, improves the heart's health

On the other hand, when we do something that seems good or morally correct, such as helping others, this emphasizes the heart's intention within our thoughts, which emphasis is duplicated in the physical heart, strengthening its function and possibly producing that "warm glow" or a similar feeling in our heart. And any other action that is an expression of the heart's intention to *reach out to those around us and spread nourishment to them*, would also have a beneficial effect on the heart. Simply talking to other people socially will do this, as will sharing our knowledge in some way.

Other effects on our speech

Our *connections with other people* are produced by the mental application of the heart's intention. And when a person has poor heart function, these connections would also tend to be poor, or "faulty". This could cause the person to have doubts about their position in society, or their worth in relation to other people, or to have other similar doubts or concerns. This may cause them to constantly try to please other people or to be inappropriately smiling and using an amused tone of voice. And since our speech is the main vehicle the heart uses to form these connections with other people, this could also cause "faults" in the person's speech, such as them speaking in inappropriate ways, making socially inept comments, or pouring out indiscriminate words—saying whatever words entered their head, to whoever would listen.

They would certainly be prone to talking too much, and could appear unable to stop talking, which may cause further social problems (further faults in their connections with other people), such as causing people to avoid their company. This would only fuel the person's insecurity, focussing their conscious mind on this "fault" in their connections with other people, causing the fault to be further duplicated in their heart's physical function, which would, in turn, only increase their tendency to adopt such behaviour—until the cycle is broken.

Poor heart function can cause dyslexia

Written words or numbers (and such things as written music) are another medium through which communication takes place, and just as with our speech, written words or numbers must have originally been devised in response to the heart's intention to *reach out to those around us and spread nourishment to them*. In other words, they are yet another expression of the heart's intention.

In patients, the start of speech defects or dyslexia can sometimes be clearly linked to disruptions in their relationships. For example, when a child's parents split up, or the child loses a parent or sibling or close friend for some other reason, the child can sometimes develop such problems. This would certainly be more so with a sensitive child, since they would be more aware of their connections with other people and therefore more affected by any disruptions in them.

The same process that produces speech defects in us, can also be responsible for making it hard for us to smoothly read words, numbers or written music. Since these faculties are also an expression of our heart's intention, any awareness we have of "faults" in our social connections (particularly in childhood) would cause those faults to be duplicated in our heart function, which, in turn, would impede our ability to smoothly read words or numbers.

If such symptoms (and the underlying poor heart function) were caused by the person's "faulty" relationships, once the relationship issues were resolved, their poor heart function would tend to eventually rectify and the speech problems or dyslexia would clear. But treating the poor heart function with acupuncture helps the person's heart to more quickly and more fully recover from the damage caused to it by the relationship issues.

Heart transplants seem to confirm the heart's mental function

Experiences reported by many heart transplant patients seem to confirm the mental and emotional functions of the heart. After their transplant, many recipients reported having new memories that appear to have come from the donor. The memories concern the donor's connections with other people, or memories of the things they loved; in other words, their emotional attachments to the things in their lives. These include preferences inherited from the donor related to food, art, music, sexual and recreational activities, and even the name of the donor's partner. Some striking examples are a young girl who received a heart transplant from a murder victim and then had such vivid memories of the victim's interaction with their murderer that these were able to be used by the police to apprehend and convict the murderer. In another case, a militant lesbian who received a heart transplant from another woman, became straight. And a vegetarian, after a heart transplant, started having irresistible cravings for meat, and meat of the particular kind that was loved by the heart donor.

Experiences of this type are so commonly reported by heart transplant patients that serious studies have been conducted of the phenomenon. In all cases, the memories contained in the implanted heart were related to the mental and emotional functions of the heart: *to reach out to other people and spread nourishment to them*; in other words, to interact with people, care for people (and things) and to form emotional attachments to them.

Improper function

Poor heart function

The *Nei Jing* authors (or their ancestors) noticed that when a patient had poor heart function (also called "Heart chi deficiency") they tended to have a selection of the signs and symptoms from list "A" below, which cleared once the heart was successfully treated. The signs and symptoms included in lists "B" to "G" below are possible complications of poor heart function. Likewise, it was noticed that when a patient had poor heart function for some time, they might also develop any of these extra signs and symptoms (along with those in list "A").

A. Palpitations; shortness of breath on exertion; spontaneous sweating; lethargy; and a weak pulse.
B. Anxiety, panic attacks, restlessness, unease; being easily startled by noises or anything unexpected in the immediate environment; speech defects such as stammering or stuttering; dyslexia; poor long-term memory; dream-disturbed sleep; insomnia.
C. Low grade fever during the day (hot flushes); night sweating; feeling a sensation of heat on the soles of the feet and palms of the hands; dry mouth, or feeling constantly thirsty.
D. Stuffiness or stabbing pains in the chest, which may radiate to the left shoulder and arm; and possibly also a blue-purple tinge to the face, lips and nails.
E. Muttering to oneself; depression or mental dullness; introverted manner, unable to make eye contact; incessant or incoherent talking; violent behaviour (hitting or scolding people); laughing and crying without reason; paranoia, hysteria, mental confusion; aphasia (partial loss of the ability to communicate with words[*]); loss of consciousness (sudden collapse or coma).
F. Chills, cold limbs; and a blue tinge to the lips.
G. Profuse sweating; feeble breathing; feeble and fading pulse; mental "cloudiness" or even coma.

Face colour, tone of voice, and food craving

It was noticed that when a patient had poor heart function, this would often produce a red complexion. Such a patient would also tend to have an amused tone of voice, as though they were constantly about to laugh, and they would tend to crave bitter food.

---

[*] There is a graphic example of this in the patient example on page 129.

Treatment

When a patient has poor heart function (has signs and symptoms from list "A" above), the following acupoints tend to become tender. When one of these acupoints is stimulated, this encourages the organ to cancel out the malfunction in itself that caused the tenderness at the acupoint, and the organ returns to normal function, so that the problem is corrected by the organ itself:

- Heart-7 (on the wrist),
- Heart-5 (on the wrist),
- Pericardium-6 (on the wrist),
- Bladder-15 (on the upper back), and
- Ren-14 (at the top of the abdomen).

The causes of poor heart function

This condition can be caused by the steadily declining heart function due to a prolonged illness (just as the function of all the organs would be affected) or, in a similar fashion, after a sudden severe disease; or it may be due to the general decline of organ functions in old age; or due to a similar weakness being inherited from our parents. It may also be caused by any of the mental or emotional factors mentioned from page 72 onwards, if these are present for a prolonged period.

In today's Chinese medicine, this condition is called "Heart chi deficiency", which is translated here as "poor heart function". In contemporary medicine, this same condition may be described using various terms, including: arrhythmia, cardiac insufficiency, coronary arteriosclerosis, angina pectoris, or general weakness.

Possible complications

The following conditions could be viewed as complications of poor heart function. In today's Chinese medicine these conditions are each given a specific term (described below), but it should be noted that none of these terms were used in the *Nei Jing* and have been adopted more recently.

Poor quality blood

When a patient has poor heart function, they might have any of the symptoms included in list "B" on page 81 above. In today's Chinese medicine, it is recognised that such patients would also usually have poor quality blood (also called "Blood deficiency"). In this case, the condition would then be called "Heart blood deficiency".

When the quality of a patient's blood becomes poor, this would usually have occurred as a result of poor function of the digestive organs, particularly the pancreas,* possibly combined with a poor diet (which itself could be a result of poor pancreas function, which produces a poor appetite and intolerances to some staple foods, such as wheat). The weakened digestive organs are then unable to manufacture blood of sufficient quality to nourish the body and organs, including the heart and the blood vessels.

Many of the symptoms in list "B" are of a mental or emotional nature. In contemporary physiology, these could be accounted for as follows.

Since the patient's blood is of poor quality (and after a while, even the tissue of the heart and blood vessels may also be affected), the heart cannot properly carry out its intention to *reach out to those around it and spreading nourishment to them*. In other words, it cannot properly nourish the other organs and tissues of the body. This heart intention is also used to process our thoughts—where it causes us to form relationships with the people around us. And since the intention of the heart is impeded in the heart organ itself (in that it cannot now properly nourish the body), the mental applica-

---

* Also called the spleen in Chinese medicine.

tion of its intention would also be impeded. It is as though our connections to the people around us are impeded, but we may not be consciously aware of why; we just feel that our connections are "faulty". And this produces the symptoms of anxiety (concern about these poor connections with the people around us, which may be of an unspecified nature), restlessness, being easily startled (by noises and anything unexpected in the surrounding environment—which we are now fundamentally uneasy about), dream disturbed sleep, poor long term memory (memory of our connections with the people in our lives, the events and so on).

Today's Chinese medicine term of "Heart blood deficiency" could be interpreted to mean: the effects that poor quality blood has on the heart. In contemporary medicine, this same condition may be described using various terms, such as: insomnia, anaemia, severe malnutrition, or depressive neuroses such as postnatal depression following haemorrhage during or after childbirth.

Treatment

Since this condition usually develops due to poor pancreas function, the main pancreas acupoints would usually be tender (due to the association between the pancreas and these acupoints), which include Pancreas-6* and Bladder-20. As usual, needling these acupoints would tend to normalize the pancreas function, which would improve the body's ability to manufacture blood. Bladder-17 (on the upper back) is often also tender in patients with poor quality blood and is therefore also frequently used in the treatment.

Since poor heart function is also present, this would also be treated, as described on page 81 above.

To treat insomnia, there is a frequently used empirical acupoint called, in Chinese, *Anmian*, which translates as:

---

* Also called Spleen-6.

"peaceful sleep". Empirical acupoints are sometimes not located on the main meridians but were found through experimentation. *Anmian* was found to become tender in some patients who suffer from insomnia, so can sometimes effectively treat insomnia.

> **Patient example**
> Female, aged 29. This patient had a history of depression and panic attacks, going back 18 months, and also suffered a wide range of other symptoms. After a few treatments, all her symptoms improved markedly. See the full case history on page 127.

How poor quality blood is diagnosed

When a patient has a number of the signs and symptoms from the following list, Chinese medicine considers them to have poor quality blood (also called "Blood deficiency"), since, theoretically, all the following signs and symptoms may be accounted for due to the organs and tissues of the body not being properly nourished; and also:

- pale complexion and lips;
- pale tongue;
- dry skin and hair, dry and withered nails, or brittle nails;
- seeing dark or light specks floating in the visual field; and
- dizziness and vertigo (due to the brain not being properly nourished).

This is a good example of the holistic approach used in Chinese medicine. There is a wide range of signs and symptoms listed above, all of which are treated by normalizing the function of the pancreas (the underlying cause) which improves the quality of the blood, so that the signs and symptoms gradually clear by themselves. The alternative approach would be to try to treat each symptom individually (for example, the dizziness, insomnia, dry skin and hair, anxiety, and so on) while leaving the function of the pancreas unchanged (the underlying cause).

In today's Chinese medicine, this condition is called "Blood deficiency"; and when this affects the heart, the combined condition is known as "Heart blood deficiency". In contemporary medicine, this same condition may be described as anaemia or malnutrition.

Internal production of heat

When tissue is damaged or stressed (such as when overworked, diseased, wounded, or deprived of nourishment for some other reason), the body produces heat at that location. And this same principle applies to the internal organs. When these are exhausted from overwork or are not properly nourished, this would cause the organ to produce heat.

In the case of patients with poor heart function, the heat produced by the stressed tissue of their heart would be experienced in the form of some, or all, of the symptoms in list "C" on page 81:

- low grade fever during the day (hot flushes);
- night sweating;
- feeling a sensation of heat on the soles of the feet and palms of the hands; and
- dry mouth, or feeling constantly thirsty.

As well as these general symptoms, the person would also be likely to experience more pronounced mental or emotional disturbances than with mere poor heart function alone (the symptoms in list "B" on page 81 above), which can be explained as follows.

Since the tissue of the heart is stressed to the point where it is producing heat, this would more severely impede the heart's intention to *reach out to those around it and spreading nour-*

ishment to them (i.e. circulate blood to nourish the organs). And this increased impediment would also be duplicated in the mental application of the heart's intention, causing an increased impediment in our connection with the people around us, which could worsen the following symptoms:

- anxiety, panic attacks, unease, restlessness, being easily startled;
- insomnia; and
- dream-disturbed sleep.

The translation of "Yin deficiency"

In today's Chinese medicine, this condition is known as "Yin deficiency". And when the heart is affected in this way, this is known as "Heart yin deficiency". In this book, I have translated "Yin deficiency" as "internal production of heat".

In contemporary medicine, this same condition (of "Heart yin deficiency") may be described using various terms, such as: arrhythmia, tachycardia, hypertension, hyperthyroidism, or anxiety neurosis.

Treatment—the body's ability to self regulate

When patients have this condition, poor heart function and probably also poor quality blood would usually have been present for some time, and the condition would be addressed by treating those underlying causes. However, the function of the other main organs is likely to also be affected (since their nourishment is impeded), producing a wide range of other signs and symptoms. But as a general rule, when the function of a single of the main organs is normalized by acupuncture treatment, the entire organ network appears to have an almost miraculous ability to self-regulate. The functions of all the organs are interrelated and therefore complex situations can sometimes develop between them, producing a wide range of signs and symptoms—on the physical, mental and emotional levels. But, perhaps due to this very interrelation, once a few of the key acupoints are needled, this appears to enable all the main organs to simply self-regulate. And after a few such treatments, patients often experience a dramatic improvement in their health, on every level. This principle applies when treating any of the main organs, not just the heart. And this self-regulatory ability tends to make the treatment of most patients straightforward*.

Stagnation of blood

When the heart function has been poor for some time, the blood may begin to stagnate. In other words the circulation becomes too sluggish. In this case, the patient would have experienced a selection of the signs and symptoms of poor heart function for some time (list "A" on page 81 above), but added to this would be the new signs and symptoms from list "D".

In today's Chinese medicine, the condition is known as "Heart blood stagnation". In contemporary medicine, the same condition may be referred to as angina pectoris, or myocardial infarction (heart attack).

Treatment

Since this condition is a complication of poor heart function, the treatment is the same as with poor heart function, only the following acupoints are often added:

- Bladder-17 (on the back), or
- Pericardium-4 (on the inner forearm).

These acupoints often become tender when the patient experiences blood stagnation. And, as with all acupoints, needling them encourages the body to clear the condition that

---

* But see page 117, regarding our mind's ability to block acupuncture treatments; and page 151, regarding the tendency of pharmaceuticals to block all natural treatments.

caused the acupoints to become tender; in other words, to normalize the blood circulation.

As with all treatments, any other organs not functioning normally would usually be treated as well. In the case of "Heart blood stagnation" and poor quality blood, this would usually include the main digestive organs (the pancreas and stomach), since they would have usually been functioning poorly for some time in order for the quality of the blood to become poor and eventually stagnated—and there would be clear signs and symptoms related to the poor function of these organs.

Mental disorders

When describing the causes of poor heart function, I said that mental or emotional states (such as those described from page 72 onwards) could sometimes impede the function of the heart. This same principle works in both directions, and sometimes extreme mental problems can be caused by poor heart function. The *Nei Jing* authors observed that patients with poor heart function could sometimes develop any of the mental symptoms from list "E" on page 81 above.

The term "phlegm"

The mechanism responsible for causing these symptoms is similar to that described under the heading: "Poor quality blood" (p.82). The poor quality blood impedes the heart's intention of *reaching out to those around it and spreading nourishment to them* (i.e. prevents the heart from properly nourishing the other organs and tissues of the body), which then correspondingly impedes the mental application of this intention, causing problems in the patient's connections with the people around them, which is at the root of many of the symptoms in list "E".

However, with the present condition, the impediment is stronger than with mere poor quality blood. When poor quality blood is present, the digestive organs (particularly the pancreas) would have functioned poorly for some time, in which case the states of *dampness* would have existed for some time (p.65). In contemporary physiology, this state could be summarized as follows. The normal excess of glucose, fats and proteins that exists in the blood shortly after eating is not properly regulated (probably mainly due to poor pancreas function), which affects the supply of nutrition to all the organs and processes, which then produces a wide range of possible signs and symptoms.

When this *dampness* has existed for some time, the poor function of the organs and systems gradually worsens, producing an increase in the number or severity of the signs and symptoms.

In today's Chinese medicine, the *dampness* would now be regarded as having transformed into *phlegm*. Simplistically, this state could be visualized as a thickening of the "soup" of excess nutrients in the blood; and since this "soup" is regarded as pathogenic (in Chinese medicine), the pathogen would now be stronger.

Hence this current condition is known in today's Chinese medicine as "Phlegm misting the mind". The meaning of this poetic term can be understood as follows. The prolonged presence of *phlegm* impedes the heart's normal function of *reaching out to those around it* (the organs and tissues) *and spreading nourishment to them*, which also prevents it from performing this same function when processing our thoughts. In other words, it severely impedes our connections with the people around us, causing the symptoms in list "E" on page 81 above. That is, the phlegm "mists our mind".

In contemporary medicine, this same condition could be referred to using a variety of terms, including: hysteria, manic and depressive psychoses, stroke sequella, aphasia, epilepsy, and in children: speech or mental retardation.

Treatment

As well as directly treating the poor heart function, the patient's main digestive organs would also be treated. When this state of *dampness* and *phlegm* has existed for some time, certain acupoints would be tender and these would usually be included in the treatment, such as Stomach-40 (on the shin).

Apart from *one or two* of the main acupoints for treating the heart and improving the digestion—such as Bladder-15 (on the upper back), Heart-7 (on the wrist), Pericardium-5 (on the wrist), Ren-14 (on the upper abdomen), Pancreas-6* (on the lower leg), or Bladder-20 (on the aback)—one of the following, more targeted, acupoints would usually also be used in this case, to assist the patient to become more clear headed:

- Du-20 (on the top of the head),
- Kidney-9 (behind the knee), or
- Gallbladder-20 (at the back of the neck).

In clinic, I find that many mental and emotional conditions can clear within a few treatments, such as anxiety, panic attacks and depression, but the speed of recovery very much depends on the underlying health of each patient. And a further large determining factor can be whether or not the patient is using strong pharmaceutical remedies. If they are, this can notably slow down the recovery time, since the patient's body no longer has chemical autonomy, therefore the ability of their main organs to self-regulate is limited (p.149).

Worsening of poor heart function

When poor heart function has been present for some time, this may gradually worsen and eventually produce the signs and symptoms in list "F" on page 81 above.

---

* Also called Spleen-6.

In today's Chinese medicine, this condition is known as "Heart yang deficiency", which can be understood as meaning a more severe case of poor heart function. When applied to an organ, the term *yang* refers to the functioning of the organ, rather than the condition of its tissue (which would be the *yin* aspect). And when the *yang* aspect (the functioning) has diminished to this level, this implies that the heart functions are themselves starting to fail. And if the condition worsens still more and becomes critical, this may produce the signs and symptoms in list "F".

Treatment

The treatment is very similar to that for poor heart function, only the use of moxibustion would usually be added (p.61). It is very unlikely that a patient's heart could have become this unwell without the function of their other main organs also being affected, and those would also be treated.

The small intestine

In contemporary physiology, the small intestine is about five meters long. It lies between the exit of the stomach and the entry to the large intestine. It fills the abdominal cavity; and the large intestine, which is about 1.5 meters long, surrounds it. The first section of the small intestine, which is about twenty-five centimetres long, is called the *duodenum*. Food from the stomach is released into this section, and the pancreas and gallbladder secrete digestive juices into the duodenum, which are combined with intestinal juices to chemically digest the food. This takes place in the walls of the small intestine, where nutrients are absorbed into the blood and lymph, which then circulate the nutrients to every part of the body.

Two thousand years ago, the *Nei Jing* authors developed theories on the role of the small intestine. But understandably, these were largely misguided. They had no notion of the small intestine playing any part in the absorption of nutrients, and regarded its role to be mainly in the elimination of waste.

The roll of the small intestine in Chinese medicine treatments

Clinically, the small intestine is not considered to be significant, which is not to say that it suffers no problems. It is extremely common for people to experience a swollen, tender or clearly dysfunctional small intestine (what has become known as IBS in contemporary medicine). However, in Chinese medicine, this is regarded as a problem related to the pancreas.

The pancreas is responsible for enabling the completion of the digestive process. In contemporary physiology, it provides the enzymes which the small intestine then uses to enable it to absorb nutrients into circulation. When a person has poor pancreas function, the secretion of these enzymes could only be inadequate in some way, which may be what prevents the small intestine from functioning properly—and the person may develop symptoms of a swollen and tender abdomen, or even loose or runny stools. Therefore, when a person has poor pancreas function they also usually suffer intestinal problems; and once the poor pancreas function is treated, the small intestine function would usually also return to normal.

It is for this reason that Chinese medicine regards the symptoms of a tender and swollen abdomen, together with loose or runny stools, as symptoms of poor pancreas function—even though they are produced by the small intestine. And when a person has these symptoms, it is their pancreas that is treated.

It should also be noted that intestinal problems are only common because poor pancreas function is extremely common. Indeed, in developed countries poor pancreas function is epidemic.

The possible mental functions

The intention of the small intestine is the same as its physical function (in contemporary physiology), which could be summarised as: *to complete the extraction of nutrients and incorporate them into circulation* (amongst those around it). As mentioned above—the physical function of the heart and small intestine are dependent on one another to be able to carry out this role. And this also applies when their functions are used to process our thoughts. But on top of this, the small intestine's close working relationship with the pancreas *also* applies in the processing of our thoughts.

The small intestine completes the digestion begun by the pancreas. The pancreas's function could be summarized as: *to further break down food* (which process the stomach began) *to find any inherent nutrition and to control the body's uptake of the main nutrition.* When this function is used to process our thoughts, this means: looking for ideas about the world around us that may be "nourishing" (ideas which might be from the media, from other people's comments, or from our own observations). The small intestine then *completes the extraction of nutrients and incorporates them into circulation* (amongst those around it). In other words, it enables the heart to perform its function of *spreading this nourishment to the people around us.* After all, if we have no ideas (no "nourishment"), we cannot spread them to other people.

To summarize, when we read or hear another person's words (for example), the stomach *begins* the process of us mentally digesting the information; and the pancreas then looks for any "nourishing" ideas amongst the words—ideas that might be suggested or implied by them, as well as any that are immediately apparent. The pancreas then absorbs these into the body (the mental equivalent perhaps being to store them in memory). The small intestine assists the pancreas to do this, by completing the extraction of these "nutrients". And both the small intestine and heart are then able to circulate any nutrients we have found—to the other people around us. By working together, they can spread the nutrients to the "body tissue" (in other words, store them in memory), or to "the other organs" (in other words, the people around us). And they do this by urging us to use some means of communication, whether it be speech, written words, eye contact, or simply body language.

When looked at in this way, the interdependence between these organs in this aspect of the processing of our thoughts seems clear. Any impediment to the stomach or pancreas function, also impedes the small intestine function, which, in turn, impedes the heart function. And conversely, when the heart function is impeded (either physically or mentally), this *also* impedes the small intestine function, exacerbating any IBS symptoms. This is because the small intestine cannot properly absorb nutrients into the blood if the blood circulation is inadequate; and also, the same mental factors that impede the heart, also impede the small intestine—as shown in the following example, which also demonstrates this interdependence.

By far the most common cause of poor pancreas function is overthinking (trying to digest too many thoughts), which usually produces in us the "small intestine" symptoms of feeling bloated and having a tender and swollen abdomen. Here, the small intestine has stopped working properly, so cannot complete the digestive process; the fabric of the organ may become inflamed, and because the food that normally passes through the small intestine cannot be processed properly by it, we may also develop loose stools. This symptom of a swollen abdomen seems to be just as common amongst men as women, only the swelling is often more severe in men. A possible explanation for this is that most societies encourage men to suppress their heart function. Men are encouraged not to share their deepest concerns, or to discuss emotional matters at all (ultimately, to live a lonely existence), which impedes their heart function (p.76). And due to the heart's interdependence with the small intestine, this would also tend to impede the small intestine function. Its function is impeded mentally—due to the reluctance to *spread nourishment to those around us*—and this impediment would be duplicated in the physical organ, weakening its function and thus exacerbating the small intestine symptoms.

The functions of all twelve organs are used to process our thoughts

It is most likely that the functions of *all* the abdominal organs are used to process our thoughts, and that the same interdependencies that exist between the physical functioning of all these organs, also exist between their functions when used to process our thoughts.

It is mainly the *yin* organs that Chinese medicine considers to have mental functions (the pancreas, liver, lungs, kidneys, and heart). They undoubtedly perform the most important roles in the processing of our thoughts, but there is no reason to think that the *yang* organs are not also utilized. With the functioning of the *physical* organs, the *yang* organs tend to service the *yin* organs in some way (they perform less important roles but roles that make it possible for the *yin* organs to perform *their* roles). And this same arrangement probably applies in the processing of our thoughts—that the functions of all twelve abdominal organs play roles which mirror the roles the organs play in the physical body—with each *yang* organ servicing its paired *yin* organ in some way.

It should be noted that all this book's arguments on the mental functions of the organs are theoretical. I have used concepts from contemporary physiology to suggest a possible explanation for this phenomena, which has always been a routine part of Chinese medicine, from the *Nei Jing* onwards. Today, the associations between our thoughts and organ functions are apparent in any Chinese acupuncture clinic, yet the concepts are alien to contemporary physiology. My suggested explanations are intended to enable today's minds to at least accept that the phenomenon may be possible.

Chapter 7. Mental and emotional factors in causing disease

From my own clinical experiences I believe it is not possible to overstate the significance of everyday mental and emotional factors in causing serious long-term disease, so I felt it worthwhile summarizing and expanding on them in this chapter.

A peculiarly human problem

The abdominal organs function in relation to each other; and the relationships between them are delicately balanced. But as humans, our conscious mind is able to readily upset this balance. How is this possible?

In evolutionary terms, the digestive organs probably existed for millions of years before creatures developed brains. Through all that time, the abdominal organs were interacting with each other to coordinate their functions. Just as happens today, this was probably achieved via nerves and chemical messengers. And in order to make these functional decisions, this network of nerves and chemical messengers must have, in effect, "had knowledge of" each organ's functions. Hence this network could be thought of as representing the logic of the organs. When the senses evolved, there is evidence that each of the senses was associated with a particular abdominal organ; and perhaps as a part of this evolutionary process, the logic of those organs was also now represented in the evolving brain (as networks of neurons and chemical messengers, just as still exist today). When we further evolved, ventured onto land and began living in complex societies, it so happens that all the new thinking and decisions that we then needed to make, could be performed by using this existing organ logic. And it is supposed that, rather than evolving new brain matter to process these new thoughts, this existing organ logic was used instead. This scenario would then explain the many similarities that exist today between the organ functions and our thoughts; and also explain the two-way causative relationships that exist between those thoughts and the signs and symptoms of malfunction in the corresponding organs, as follows.

When our mind uses the organ logic to process our thoughts, and our conscious mind suppresses, overuses, or is aware of the impeding of particular thoughts, this situation is duplicated in the related physical organ, which causes that organ to act as though its physical functions had been suppressed, overused, or impeded. This upsets the delicate balance between the organs, which took millions of years to evolve, and the organs become stressed, which causes them to produce the signs and symptoms of our illness (see *Acupuncture Today and in Ancient China* for more detail).

The effect on the main organs

Pancreas and stomach

In contemporary physiology, the stomach starts the process of digestion, and the pancreas acts *to further break down food to find any inherent nutrition and to control the body's uptake of the main nutrition.* In our mental world, our thoughts take the place of physical food; and the functions of the stomach and pancreas are used to digest those thoughts.

In developed societies today, we tend to think all day long—in our work, studies, recreation, or in simply trying to understand the apparently puzzling people around us. Therefore our conscious mind overuses the pancreas and stomach, which become weakened through overuse.

Significantly, the thoughts we most often strive to digest are those that are hard to understand. The physical equivalent would be to choose the hardest to digest food and to eat this difficult food all day long. And when we are unable to properly digest any particular thought, this *failure to digest* is duplicated in the pancreas, causing it to tend to fail to digest physical food. It is as though the normal physical food were transformed into hard-to-digest food by the action of our mind. And when our mind does this for most of the day, year after year, it eventually renders the pancreas no longer able to properly digest normal food.

To make matters worse, the pancreas function peaks at eleven a.m., which is when the normal digestive ability is at its strongest. From this time onwards, the pancreas function weakens as the day progresses. Yet our conscious mind continues heavily using this digestive ability all day long, which only weakens it even further. With physical food, once we have eaten enough, we are "full" and we normally stop eating; yet because it is our mind doing the digesting, we think it is okay to push ourselves to "eat" more and more thoughts, even though we may have the same feeling of being "full", of having "eaten" enough thoughts for the moment. If we were to do this with physical food and push ourselves to go on eating all day long, no-one would be surprised at the resultant symptoms of ill health. But we consider our mind to be separate from the body, and so do not normally make the connection between thinking too much and suffering the symptoms that would inevitably result from eating hard-to-digest food and doing this all day long.

The usual physical symptoms are: feeling tired and bloated after eating, having a swollen and tender abdomen, loose stools, intolerances to foods such as dairy and wheat, a poor sense of taste, low energy in general, and a sluggish mind (p.14). All such symptoms tend to be common amongst students, in people whose work requires them to think intensively, and people who habitually worry. And the more a person becomes exhausted through overthinking, the more pronounced these symptoms become. In particular, their ability to think would worsen. This is because the relationship between an organ's physical and mental functions is reciprocal, and once a person has poor pancreas function, their ability to mentally digest information also becomes poor. They would tend to get stuck in endless cycles of thought, unable to reach a satisfactory conclusion (that is, become unable to properly digest thoughts), which would usually result in them working their digestion even harder.

Added to the above symptoms can sometimes be a feeling of indigestion; that is, a cramping feeling on the front, left side of the torso (the location of the stomach). Often, with people whose digestion is already weakened through overthinking, when they are unable to *begin* digesting a particular thought, they experience this cramping feeling in their stomach—as though they had swallowed some physical food that their stomach could not digest.

Liver

In contemporary physiology, the liver regulates the production and supply of energy and the circulation of blood and other resources to the organs and tissues of the body. This could be summarized as: *to monitor the flow of substances to the organs and tissues, and when this does not seem right, to regulate the flow.*

When this function is used to process our thoughts, it is those thoughts that become the mental equivalent of the energy and substances in the body, and it so happens that our conscious mind often notices things that *do not seem right* in our thoughts, which then obstructs the flow of our thoughts. When this happens, this causes the liver to act as though the flow of the energy and substances in the body had been obstructed, so it applies its regulatory ability to attempt to remove the obstruction. It does this creatively, and (just as it does in the body with the supply of energy and other resources) it rearranges our thoughts, swaps or compares them with our memories (our reserve resources) until it has transformed the thought so as to remove the problem that was obstructing its flow.

This creative ability causes the liver to produce countless "rules" about how things should be done, and is responsible for us being able to efficiently organize the world around us and also every aspect of our own and other people's behaviour. Indeed, much of the organization that makes society function would not be possible without the liver's creative ability—such as the ordering of the day into time slots, and the ordering of every activity into an efficient process, right down to the smallest of the routine tasks we perform.

However, this causes a problem for us when other people, or other things, do not behave exactly as we would like them to (when they break our "rules"). This obstructs the flow of our thoughts, which causes the liver to behave as though the flow of the energy and substances in the body had been obstructed. In response, it usually resorts to its emergency measure of producing a powerful force to remove the obstruction—the emotion of anger. We might express this by sighing or we may simply suppress our anger. But after a while, this suppressed anger builds up until we can no longer contain it, when we might start shouting to attempt to force people to do what we want; or we may even resort to physical violence to get our will obeyed (and the obstruction removed), which accounts for such things as road rage attacks and most relationship hostility—be it at home, work, or socially.

In all of us, this process is responsible for the daily stress-related symptoms we suffer—when our train is late, traffic moves too slowly, a queue is too long, or our employer expects us to produce several hour's work in one hour, or do the job of three people all at once. All these situations obstruct the physical function of the liver, which could eventually produce symptoms such as: moodiness, depression, irritability, rage, migraines, insomnia; stiff neck, shoulders and other joints; muscular cramps and spasms; painful periods, premenstrual syndrome; and also many other possible symptoms related to poor circulation, poor energy and poor digestion—which are indirect effects of the liver function being obstructed.

Due to the reciprocal nature of the relationship between an organ's mental and physical functions, once a person develops stagnated liver function, the mental application of their liver function would tend to become overactive—reflecting the liver's desire to remove the stagnation. In our mental world, the liver does this by applying its creative ability; or enforcing the countess "rules" this ability previously worked out; or frequently resorting to its emergency measure of producing anger. The person would become over controlling and excessively organized, would angrily insist on other people strictly obeying all rules; and would also tend to be paranoid.

The production of paranoia

Since the liver's creative ability is the key method it uses to remove an obstruction, when our conscious mind sees obstructions everywhere (our "rules" not being obeyed by people), the liver's creative ability is over applied to social situations, which tends to produce paranoia, as follows.

The liver would use its creative ability to try to work out why a person was behaving in a strange way, or was doing something that *we* thought was wrong. And it so happens that when someone else's behaviour is analysed from *our* point of view, it is easy to interpret their words, actions, tone of voice or facial expressions as indicating malicious intent towards ourselves. And this is the solution the liver would usually come up with, which it then presents to our conscious mind—the idea that the person was behaving maliciously towards us. Hence the liver has removed the obstruction to the flow of our thoughts—since the person's behaviour now makes sense to us.

But this would then usually cause the liver to also create countermeasures for us to adopt against this person, to, again, remove this further (now self-created) obstruction—the new obstruction being the notion that this person was breaking the rules of social conduct by behaving maliciously towards us. Our creative countermeasure would be designed to harm the other person. This might be a scheme to undermine them in other people's eyes, with carefully planned actions; or simply the making of malicious comments of our own. Though our behaviour would make perfect sense to us, it would only seem puzzling to the other person, since this further obstruction was imaginary (they were *not* behaving maliciously, so our response would make no sense to them). And the more the liver perceives such obstructions to the flow of our thoughts, the more it strives to find such creative solutions (now perhaps trying to imagine an explanation for why the "malicious" person was denying behaving in that way), and the more tormented we become.

The downside of creative ability

The ability to produce creative thoughts is an accidental offshoot of the liver's regulatory function. When our mind uses this simple liver function, which was designed to regulate the flow of substances and energy in the body, the function is, in effect, transformed into a creative engine that shapes our mental world. When used to process our ever-present thoughts, this creative ability goes rampant (since our thoughts are such that the obstructions to their flow are rampant), and it creates countless "rules" which are stored in our memory and *only* apply to our own particular mental world.

This massive collection of rules then creates advantages for us—enabling us to organize, to invent, to learn many skills. But these same rules also create a massive potential for obstructing the function of our physical liver—since all these rules must be obeyed for our liver to act as though the substances and energy in our body were flowing correctly.

How does the liver know when something is not right in our thoughts?

In the body, when the flow of energy or other resources is impeded, this would usually be because one or more of the organs were not functioning properly—due to their own functions being impeded for some reason. When the liver function is used to process our thoughts, it follows that the same must be true. Our thoughts are present amongst the logic of all the organs (just as the energy and substances are present amongst all the physical organs), and the flow of these thoughts would usually be impeded when the logic (mental function) of any of the main organs becomes impeded, which would usually happen due to it being unable to process a particular thought.

For example, the pancreas may be unable to digest a particular thought, or the lungs unable to find quality in the thought, or the kidneys may notice that the thought threatens our survival or status (the thought may undermine us socially or at work, or suggest we participate in conduct or a venture that is financially or physically reckless), or the heart may notice that the thought demonstrates poor social connections (it may be treating someone unfairly, unjustly or inappropriately). Any such situation would cause the flow of our thoughts to be impeded, which is the cue for the liver to act to "regulate the flow", since "something does not seem right" in the flow. The liver's creative ability would then attempt to modify the thought to remove the obstruction. It may rely on remembered solutions or rearrange the thought while perhaps combining it with other remembered thoughts, so as to create a new thought that solved the problem—just as the liver creatively manages the body's resources and energy to remove physical obstructions: by interchanging them when necessary, calling on reserves to solve a shortfall, creating new energy, such as ATP, and so on. At this point the thought may be digested (since it now makes sense); or its quality may be improved (the process, action, or appearance of an object or person now seems right); or the thought may now reflect a proper social connection (the other person is now being treated justly, fairly, or appropriately); or the new thought may no longer be too risky for us. This would pacify the "complaining organ" and thus restore the flow of our thoughts. And the liver would no longer have reason to act as though the flow of energy and substances in the body were obstructed—so would no longer produce the emotion of irritation or anger. And, indeed, the energy and substances in the body *would* return to flowing properly.

Lungs

In contemporary physiology, the lungs extract oxygen from the air we breathe and expel the waste products of respiration, which could be summarized as: *to take in something intangible from outside us, sort the good from the bad, incorporate the precious and let go of the waste.* When this lung logic is used to process our thoughts it enables us to notice quality in the things around us, to incorporate this within ourselves—so we are enriched through the appreciation of quality—and to *let go of the waste*; that is, to stop caring about something that is harmful to us, to let go of it and move on.

When our mind applies this logic in a balanced way, this enables us to gain pleasure from such things as music, nature, architecture, fashion, or design in any area, such as in electronic gadgets, cars, furniture, and so on. This also applies to personalities; we gain pleasure from the quality we recognise in certain people, in the way they conduct themselves, morally, physically, verbally. And the other aspect of this mental activity of *sorting the good from the bad* is that it enables us to recognise poor quality in all these things—in music, fashion, architecture, design, and in personalities. In other words, to recognise the opposite of what *we* personally think of as "quality". And once this "waste" has been sorted, if the lung function is healthy, we are able to *let go of the waste*, which enables us to let go of something harmful to us. As well as general "poor quality" experiences, this could also include activities, tasks or relationships that we have begun but which have become harmful rather than rewarding.

Our appreciation of quality can clearly greatly enrich our lives. But further than this, each time we appreciate quality in something, this strengthens the lung function. When our conscious mind uses this lung logic, and something precious from the things we experience is successfully extracted, this success is duplicated in the lungs and enhances the lungs' ability to extract oxygen from the air we breathe. This is why, when we experience something we enjoy, such as a landscape, fine piece of music or good design in any area, we may feel we can breathe more easily and may even sigh with pleasure.

However, when our conscious mind overuses this lung function we become perfectionists and inevitably end up living in an almost constant state of disappointment. The more we focus on quality, the higher our standards become and the less we are able to find it. This constant failure to extract something precious from the things we experience is duplicated in the lungs; and the lungs' ability to extract oxygen from the air we breathe is impeded. In time, this tendency could weaken the lung function, producing such symptoms as: shortness of breath, a weak cough, a quiet and weak voice, poor energy, the tendency to suffer colds and flu, a poor sense of smell, a blocked nose and sinuses, and wheezing or asthma—where it is difficult to breathe out (p.40).

Once a person develops poor lung function (either through mental factors or physical disease), their lungs' mental functions would also be poor. Their lungs' ability to breathe out and expel the waste products of respiration (CO_2) would be poor, so that the person's mental ability to *let go of the waste* would also be poor and they would tend to continue with projects, activities, habits, relationships, long after they had become harmful to them. And their lungs' ability to extract the precious oxygen from the air they breathe would also be poor, so that their ability to mentally *sort the good from the bad* would be poor. They would find it harder to appreciate quality in the things they experience, which would only increase further their tendency to be a perfectionist; for the lungs' ability to extract oxygen from the air we breathe is an essential and urgent urge (if we cannot extract oxygen, we will die) and once this is impeded, this urgent urge would be duplicated in the mental aspect of the lung function, driving us all the more to seek quality—with the quiet desperation of an animal trying to breathe air that is starved of oxygen. But since our ability to appreciate quality would be weak, we would feel dissatisfied with most things and end up living in a constant state of sadness.

Heart

In contemporary physiology, the heart circulates nourishment to the other organs and to every tissue via the blood vessels, which could be summarized as: *reaching out to those around us and spreading nourishment to them.* When this function is used to process our thoughts, this produces in us the desire to share our knowledge with those around us, or to help or assist them, which is all done most readily by talking to them—which reflects the fact that speech, and our facility with language, is the sense associated with the heart. And whenever we act on these desires and help other people or simply talk to them, this successful application of the heart's intention is duplicated in the heart, which enhances its physical function—sometimes to the extent that it produces that "warm glow" feeling within it.

However, our mind can also impede the heart function. In most societies this happens most commonly in men, who are encouraged not to talk about personal matters or their feelings, and to deal with things alone, without complaining or seeking assistance from others. When thinking in such ways, the heart's intention is suppressed in our thoughts, which state is duplicated in the heart, suppressing its physical function and also undermining the circulatory system.

The heart function can also be impeded in other situations, such as whenever a social connection is broken, which happens whenever a friendship, association, or relationship ends. The physical pain we feel in the heart reflects the degree to which the heart function is impeded, which can happen to such a degree that people can sometimes literally die of a "broken heart". A long-term relationship ends, or a job they held and loved for many years ends, and the break in that particular social connection is so severe that their heart can no longer function and simply stops working; that is, they suffer a heart attack.

When the heart function is routinely impeded and becomes weakened, this can eventually produce symptoms such as: palpitations, shortness of breath on exertion, anxiety or panic attacks, restlessness, being easily startled, speech disorders or dyslexia, having a poor long term memory, dream-disturbed sleep, insomnia, spontaneous sweating, lethargy, stabbing pains or "stuffiness" in the chest, possibly culminating in a heart attack (p.80).

Once a person develops poor heart function (either due to mental factors or physical disease), their heart's mental functions would also be poor, or "faulty". And since the mental application of their heart function produces their connections with other people, these would also be "faulty". They may habitually make socially inappropriate comments, behave in socially unacceptable ways, be constantly trying to please other people or inappropriately smiling and using an amused tone of voice. Every aspect of their interaction with other people could seem inappropriate.

Kidneys

In contemporary physiology, the "kidneys" (which includes three structures: the kidneys, adrenal glands and gonads) are responsible for a wide range of functions concerned with ensuring our immediate and long-term survival. This includes assisting in the regulation of our energy, releasing reserves to cope with emergency situations (the adrenaline surge), supporting and enabling immunity, and all functions related to reproduction.

When this logic is used to process our thoughts, this produces in us motivations and ideas related to our long-term survival, which includes us setting goals in life, having the drive to pursue them, and also the will to go on living. And the kidneys also generate defensive thoughts (such as the protective lies that seem to spontaneously pop into our mind when we are threatened), and also opportunistic thoughts that favour us (such as the idea to commit an opportunistic theft, or to act in some way or say something that favours us in the eyes of our boss or a potential partner).

The kidney function is most often weakened by overuse of the reserves the kidneys call upon in times of emergency. In the modern world, instead of this being restricted to truly emergency situations, such as when our life is physically threatened, it is more usual for us to draw on these reserves merely to achieve demanding tasks, or to keep functioning when the body is tired, causing us to live in an almost constant state of "emergency". This is most common in the workplace, but it also happens socially, recreationally and in family life. We are driven to work too hard, often through fear or ambition, but also sometimes through sheer excitement—which is just as harmful for the kidneys. Living in an almost constant adrenalized state overuses this kidney function and eventually weakens the kidneys, producing various symptoms which could include: low back pain, shortness of breath, asthma (where it is hard to breathe in), the tendency to suffer hay fever and other allergies; migraines, feeling constantly fearful, having a poor short term memory and concentration, frequent urination, weak knees and stiff joints generally, poor hearing, low libido and decreased engagement in life (p.59).

The kidneys also regulate the production and use of energy, support immunity and provide us with the urge to want to be alive and continue living. Our hopes, ambitions, or our own awareness of our status are all ideas produced in us when the kidney logic is used to process our thoughts. When any of these ideas are dashed, this impedes this kidney logic, which impediment is duplicated in the physical kidneys. Apart from contributing to any of the above symptoms, this could also remove our will to live, greatly reduce our energy, immunity, and possibly cause a long term depression. It is as though the body's drive were switched off.

Another mental cause of poor kidney function is when a person routinely feels fearful, vulnerable or unsupported. These feelings undermine our long-term survival, and since the kidney logic produces our thoughts concerning our long-term survival, this undermines the kidneys' logic and hence also their physical function.

This mental state is common in the modern world. Concerns about being able to pay the bills, pay the rent or mortgage, or about remaining in employment, or in a relationship—are common preoccupations for many people. And such fears are epidemic amongst men. Indeed, the self-imposed loneliness that society encourages men to adopt, tends to foster a feeling of being unsupported, which would cause feelings of fearfulness and insecurity, leading to poor kidney function, with its related signs and symptoms. This would then tend to worsen the situation, since the fear and insecurity would only increase (one of the possible symptoms of poor kidney function is an increased tendency to feel fearful). And the more the kidney reserves were further drawn on—to combat this threat to our survival—the more the kidney function would be weakened.

The interdependence of the organs when processing our thoughts

Just as the functioning of the physical organs is interdependent, this also applies when the organ logic is used to process our thoughts, and many of the daily tasks we perform require the combined use of the logic of all the main organs.

For example, the single task of researching something on the internet or in a reference book would require us to digest information (a pancreas function), an element of creative thinking (a liver function), attention to quality and the discarding of "waste" (a lung function), processing of other people's words and composing some of our own, to be either written or spoken (a heart function), and the task may have been motivated by us wanting to enhance our value in the eyes of other people, either with a long- or short-term goal in mind (a kidney function).

We are so used to the experience of our mental daily lives that we take it for granted and simply assume all tasks are performed by the brain which is some sort of massive computer. It is not until each task is broken down, as in the above example, that it becomes clear that our mental world is, in fact, made up by combining the mental functions of all the abdominal organs.

The downside of this is that, since the functions of all the main organs are usually utilized when we perform many tasks, all the organs can be affected when a task becomes stressful.

For example, in many work-related scenarios, there is pressure for us to do tasks in too short a time. This would impede the liver function, since the situation would be seen by the liver's logic as the breaking of our "rules". This would produce stress-related symptoms within us, and in particular, irritation and anger. But the lung function would also be impeded, since our desire for quality was disappointed. It is the lungs that enable us to appreciate the quality in abstract things, such as doing a good job, and when we are conscious of such quality being sacrificed, this impedes the lung's logic and hence also its physical function. And the kidney function could also be weakened, since if we did not do our job well, we might fear losing our job and then not being able to survive, which would undermine the part of the kidneys' logic concerned with our long-term survival, and thus weaken the kidneys' physical function. And we might also be inclined to draw on our emergency reserves to counter this and meet the demands of our job, which would only further weaken the kidneys. And if we did not have good social bonds at work (with supervisors and others—perhaps as a result of the stress), the heart function would also be impeded—possibly producing in us that "sinking heart" feeling whenever we thought of our work environment. And in many jobs, the work itself may also be depleting for the pancreas (even without the stress), since it is the pancreas and stomach that enable us to mentally digest information. And since we were employed for eight hours a day, we would be expected to be mentally digesting information for this whole time, even though our ability to do this peaks at eleven a.m., and weakens from then onwards as the day progresses. This forced overuse would greatly weaken the pancreas function. But also, we would usually be attempting to digest hard-to-understand thoughts (the equivalent of difficult-to-digest food), which would add a further strain on the pancreas.

In all, these common work-related stresses could eventually produce in us signs and symptoms related to the poor function of all the main organs.

Our personality choices can impede the organ functions

Living in a human society is a complex task, and usually we must each use our own initiative to solve the problem of how to be a human being. Through years of experimentation, we make many decisions about how we should conduct ourselves in our daily lives, and these choices may also suppress the function of the main organs.

For example, there may be complex reasons why many of us sometimes avoid giving to charity. The liver creates countless "rules" and insists they are obeyed (by ourselves as well as by others); the kidneys are concerned with safeguarding our own survival; and the lungs appreciate quality—in the conduct of other people as well as in ourselves. All these desires, when combined, might cause us to develop a whole range of reasons why we should not give to charity. If our rules were broken by the person in need (perhaps simply by the fact that they were begging), or by the advertising that sought help on their behalf (such as when advertisers use emotionally manipulative devices to prompt us to support their cause); or if helping the other person could in any way threaten our own survival—all these factors could cause us to suppress the heart function of *reaching out to the other person and spreading nourishment to them.* And if we did this routinely, this would only impede our own heart function.

As another example—if we allowed the "concerns" of the lungs to dominate our mental world and tended to focus too much on quality, this may cause us to notice the poor quality in other people's responses when we talked to them. For example, when making a comment we might notice they usually misinterpreted it, or seemed incapable of understanding it in the way we meant it; or each time we started to say something, a particular person might always try to anticipate what we were saying (but clearly getting it wrong) and so would never let us finish what we started to say. When we notice such poor quality, we may stop trying to talk to people in general, which would suppress the heart's intention (to *reach out to them and spread nourishment to them*) and thus impede its physical function. And this situation may also cause us to give up on pursuits or goals in life, feeling there was no point attempting to interact with people, which would impede the kidney function (which produces our engagement with life, activities and people), and the resulting low spirits, sadness and melancholy would also impede all the other organs and bodily functions—all resulting from us focusing *too* much on quality.

As yet another example—we may have decided it was not appropriate to defend ourselves against certain injustices, perhaps in the workplace (injustices that the hierarchy demands we silently endure), or injustices in our daily interactions with friends and acquaintances—because it seemed to us unseemly to complain about such things. In all these instances, these types of injustice would be experienced by the liver as the breaking of its "rules" (because the people were not behaving as *we* believed they should), and the liver would produce anger to attempt to remove these obstructions to the flow of our thoughts. But since we had decided not to respond, this decision would also suppress our anger, producing stagnated liver function and making us prone to outbursts of anger (when we could no longer contain it) and other powerful symptoms, such as a stiff neck, muscular cramps, sciatica, abdominal or back pains, migraines, paranoia, painful periods in women.

Some people may even adopt a general policy of not defending themselves, since it seems to them improper in some way; in effect, they have decided to adopt the role of the martyr and to silently endure injustices inflicted on them by other people, because this response (or lack of it) seems to them more noble or more worthy in some other way. In this situation, not only would their liver be affected as described above, but the function of their immune system could also be impeded, since their conscious mind had decided to suppress their defences—which could affect the function of their pericardium or lymphatic system, and possibly also the aspects of their "kidneys" and lungs involved in immunity.

Acupuncture normalizes the mental functions of the organs

Acupuncture treatment seems to "get under the radar" of our conscious mind and return the physical organ functions to normal, which then also tends to regulate the mental functions of those organs. In the first few weeks of treatments, new patients often tell me of the mental changes they have spontaneously made in their lives. They might say they are less affected by things, or do not let things get to them like they used to; that they have started standing up for themselves, which makes them feel good; or they make other such comments.

The mind can block treatment

But in these first few weeks of treatment, some patients sometimes re-establish their previous mental habits, and the symptoms they were suffering start to return. For example, if a patient's liver function was stagnated for years, once this was treated they would be less inclined to mentally over-control everything in their lives—since their liver would now be functioning normally and therefore the flow of energy and substances in their body would not be obstructed, so their liver would be less inclined to control those substances. And this relaxation of control would usually be duplicated in their mental world. But if they had a long-term habit of controlling and organizing themselves and others, they may simply continue the habit—even though their physical liver was no longer experiencing obstructions. And just as before, their attempts to control and organize would often be either resisted or unsuccessful, and this obstructed state would be duplicated in their physical liver, re-establishing its stagnated function. When this happens, all the related symptoms would return and the old pattern would be re-established.

In this situation, the person's mental habits would have blocked the acupuncture treatment. With such patients, they tend to initially respond to treatment, with their symptoms being alleviated, but then after a few treatments they re-establish their mental patterns; and each treatment from then onwards has little effect on their symptoms, or the effects only last for a day or two before the symptoms return. This type of mental factor makes it harder to treat some patients and is the biggest *natural* block to acupuncture treatment.[1] The only way for such patients to improve their health would be to find some way to persuade themselves to change their mental habits—or to resist re-establishing them after treatment.

Our mental world is produced by the abdominal organs

In humans, the functions of the abdominal organs are now used to process our thoughts, so that our "mental" world was made possible because of the existence of our abdominal organ functions. Therefore our mental world is a reflection, or ghost, of our "organ" world. And because of the association between each organ's logic and its physical function, what happens in our mental world is duplicated in our organ world—and vice versa—so that each has become a model of the other.

This gives our mind the ability to cause serious physical illness

The organs were designed to do particular physical tasks, and our mental world is produced (accidentally) by this same processing. Hence, the liver provides us with the capacity to control and organize; the lungs, the capacity to appreciate quality; the pancreas, the ability to digest information; and the heart, the desire to help others. Such activities can be intoxicating and it is all too easy to fall into the habit of overusing a particular organ's processing ability—and becoming too controlling, too much of a perfectionist, a heavy thinker, or being too giving. When we do this, this causes problems for that particular abdominal organ, which is also overused; and sometimes its function my become blocked (just as its associated mental processing often meets obstructions). When these types of problems occur, it is this that causes many of the signs and symptoms of our illness.

This situation has created one of the biggest hazards for our health. If our mental world were separate from our "organ world", there would be no problem, but the two cannot be separated; what happens in the one is duplicated in the other. This means that the human intellect is a mechanism that can easily and very effectively impede the function of any, or all, of the abdominal organs. We cannot *un*-invent our intellect (that is what makes us human), so to achieve a healthy and happy life, we need to apply that intellect to regulate our own mental world, so that we do not undermine our very foundations—the functioning of our organs.

Avoiding thought patterns that impede our organ functions

On page 114 above, an example was given of the stresses we encounter in a typical work-related scenario, where there was pressure to do tasks in too short a time, and our response to that stress affected the five main organs. This is a situation many of us frequently find ourselves in. Indeed this type of scenario is almost unavoidable; these situations may draw us in, unsuspecting, until we find ourselves trapped into adopting such self-destructive mental habits.

One approach to avoiding the build up of such stress is to make adjustments in small steps. For example, many liver-related issues could be summarized as us trying to control too many things. In the tasks we routinely perform at home or at work, the liver would have worked out the most efficient process to do each task, and the liver produces in us the feeling of irritation or anger when we watch someone else doing it differently or if someone presses *us* to do it differently. Once our conscious mind is in the habit of overusing this liver function, it is easy to fill our days with endless things that must be organized or done in a very specific way, and to become entrapped into impeding our own liver function—which happens each time any of these tasks is *not* performed exactly as we would like. The particular way we would like each task performed is a "rule" our liver has created. If we could persuade ourselves to not care about such "rules" (particularly the ones other people routinely break), then the rules would go away and there would be less opportunities for the liver function to be impeded. With each such task, you could try asking yourself: is this really necessary? Can it be left out? What would happen if I did not do this at all, or in this particular way?

It is also easy to develop the habit of overusing the lung function of appreciating quality and to become entrapped into seeking ever higher standards in every aspect of our life, causing us to work excessively hard to meet our own high standards and to reject many things we might otherwise have been able to enjoy. One solution may be to try focusing on the good aspects of anything we encounter, rather than the bad; and each time we are able to appreciate something we might otherwise have rejected, the experience becomes enjoyable and our lung function is reinforced, rather than being impeded due to us failing to perceive "quality" in the things around us.

Our need to digest information will always be present, but the depleting effect on the pancreas could best be reduced by, where possible, reducing the amount of thinking (or worrying) we do and only processing the thoughts that are really "necessary". And when heavy thinking *is* necessary, if this were restricted to the morning, before about midday (the digestion peaks at eleven a.m.), this would reduce the depleting effect.

The best way to avoid weakening the kidney function would usually be to adjust our work-life balance. It is okay (and even desirable) to sometimes work hard, but this should be balanced by rest and relaxation. There should be an equal balance of activities in our life between work and play (activities that are purely enjoyable and have no element of stress). And of course the most relaxing activity we can perform is sleep. This is necessary to allow the body to repair itself. If you find yourself working hard too often and not allowing enough time each day for relaxation, or purely enjoyable activities, then you could try asking yourself what would happen if you did less. If you work hard to buy particular possessions or holidays, would you have a better overall quality of life if you modified those ambitions? If you were currently driven by the fear of unemployment or the loss of your current status, would you really be worse off if you changed your job, or might that lead to an improvement in your quality of life? And another important factor concerning kidney health is to ensure that our goals and ambitions are appropriate and achievable.

To enhance the health of our heart, we need to avoid thoughts that weaken our connections with other people; or find ways to strengthen those connections. The heart's intention is to *reach out to those around us and spread nourishment to them*. There are complex reasons why men (for example) tend to impeded this heart function. Peer pressure may inhibit men from being open about their feelings or from asking for assistance from other people. In such situations, for us to allow ourselves to share or express our opinions or feelings, it may be necessary to question the validity of the pressures that restrict us. These pressures are always self-created; it is our own response to the people around us (or our response to our own perceptions) that produces the pressure within us to keep silent, which only damages our own heart. But these types of issue are complex, and some experimentation may be required for each person to find the approach that works best for them—when every factor of their life is considered. It is often not easy to be a human being and it can take many years into adulthood (or sometimes decades) before we have become reasonably skilful at it.

Achieving the right balance in life

In our mental world, there should be a certain amount of organization, of us setting and following rules, seeking quality, thinking, having regard for others, and also watching out for our own security. The key is to get the balance right, to do each thing in proportion—to the right amount and at the right time.

A person who achieves this would always be able to "sort the good from the bad" and "let go of the waste", so they appreciate the good qualities in people (including themselves) and in all other things, without paying undue attention to minor flaws. They would also not fall into the trap of becoming *too* organized and regimented, would be able to relax rules when appropriate and allow things to happen in their own way, rather than trying to control all people and all things around them. They would not think *too* much and end up constantly mulling over every detail of their lives, the people in it, and every activity, object or idea they encountered. They would not seek too high a quality in all things and all people, so they ended up rejecting much they would otherwise benefit from. They would be able to form social connections appropriately and provide support and "nourishment" to others when appropriate, while not falling into the trap of doing this excessively. They would have formed long- and short-term goals that were achievable, rather than destroying themselves in the pursuit of goals that were not realistically achievable. And they would feel the appropriate amount of fear and excitement and sadness and anger in the appropriate situations, but not feel any of these excessively.

Observing seasonal changes

Another important element in the mental causes of disease is the disharmony with the seasons that life in today's devolved countries tends to encourage. The human body is still very much synchronized with nature. As one season changes to another, the functional balance between the organs also naturally changes. The organs find this transition demanding, which is why there tends to be epidemics of colds and influenza as each season changes. Leading up to the change, people are often drained due to driving themselves too hard; and as the season changes, this places even more demands on their organs, to the point where they are unable to maintain normal immunity and they succumb to colds and influenza. Epidemics at these times are mainly due to this effect, which is why they occur at *every* seasonal change, not only the change between Autumn and Winter—though this particular change is most demanding on our immunity, since the change is from lung-dominant to kidney-dominant, so that both the organs involved in our immunity are taxed. This explains why even more people tend to succumb at this time, and particularly the elderly, whose kidney function is often poor anyway.

When people have acupuncture treatment routinely (even if only once or twice a season), this tends to make them much more aware of their body and they can usually clearly feel the effect on themselves as the functional balance between their organs changes to prepare them for each new season. Usually they describe feeling a dramatic drop in their energy, with no apparent cause, which lasts for one or two days before their energy returns to normal and they feel subtly different. For all the above reasons, it is important to properly relax in the week when each season changes (see the tables below).

The body's resources also vary with the seasons. The Spring and Summer are the times of maximum energy, when new projects should be started and we can work hard at achieving our goals. In the Autumn and Winter our energy is naturally declining, and we should not expect to be able to work so hard. In the Winter our productivity may be about half of that in the Summer, or even less. The Winter is a time of hibernation, when our working day should be much shorter (even if present in the workplace, our productivity should be much less) and we should not start new, demanding projects. Only by living in harmony with these seasonal changes can we expect to maintain good health. And conversely, if we fail to observe the seasonal changes at all, we should expect our health to suffer.

When referring to the dates in the following tables, it should be noted that not all people adjust to each new season on the same day. With each person, the exact day their body adjusts could occur several days (or even more than a week) on either side of the following dates.

The seasonal cycle of organ activity

Table 1. The seasons in the Northern hemisphere

Approximate dates	Season	Dominant organ
21 Mar (vernal equinox) to 20 Jun	Spring	liver
21 Jun (summer solstice) to 21 Sep	Summer	heart
22 Sep (autumnal equinox) to 21 Dec	Autumn (Fall)	lungs
22 Dec (winter solstice) to 20 Mar	Winter	"kidneys"

The pancreas is not included in the above table, since the season in which its function dominates is unclear. From my own experience, it seems that the last three to four weeks of each season acts as a transitional period and that the pancreas is the dominant organ in each of these transitional periods. Also note that the body adjusts to this transitional period, just as it does to the start of each new season.

Table 2. The seasons in the Southern hemisphere

Approximate dates	Season	Dominant organ
21 Mar (autumnal equinox) to 20 Jun	Autumn (Fall)	lungs
21 Jun (winter solstice) to 21 Sep	Winter	"kidneys"
22 Sep (vernal equinox) to 21 Dec	Spring	liver
22 Dec (summer solstice) to 20 Mar	Summer	heart

Chapter notes

[1] Pharmaceutical intervention is not a natural phenomenon, so is not considered here. Once a patient is taking strong pharmaceuticals, so that their body no longer has chemical autonomy, all natural healing would be impeded to some degree. This usually produces an unclear symptom picture in the patient (one that does not resemble the patterns observed over

thousands of years in Chinese medicine), and any improvements in organ function which the acupuncture treatment produces may lapse after a day or two. This effect is similar to the "re-programming" effect that a patient's mind has when the patient stubbornly continues harmful mental habits despite the acupuncture treatment normalizing their physical organ functions. After a few days, the old pattern of organ malfunction would start to re-establish. The difference between this and the effect of pharmaceuticals, is that the patient whose treatment is being blocked by their own insistence on repeating harmful mental habits, would still have a clear symptom picture that makes perfect sense in Chinese medicine. However, their "mental block" to treatment would make permanent progress in their treatment challenging.

Chapter 8. Detailed case histories

With many patients it is common for them to have signs and symptoms relating to all five of their main organs (as in most of the following case histories). This probably reflects the fact that the organs are interdependent, so that once a problem exists in one for any length of time, the other main organs are inevitably affected.

In the case histories, I mention which organ malfunctions are responsible for causing the various signs and symptoms, but do not usually state which acupoints were used in the treatments and instead only record the general progress of the treatments. The typical acupoints used to treat each organ can be found in the chapters related to those organs.

Depression and panic attacks

Female, aged 29. This patient initially sought treatment for depression and panic attacks. She had a history of depression and mild panic attacks, going back 18 months, and recently suffered a severe panic attack. Following an argument with her boyfriend, she started to feel panicky in the street; she was hyperventilating, started to feel faint, felt cramp in the fingers of both hands, but more so on her left, and also cramp around her jaw and she was unable to speak. Apart from these attacks, she also had the following symptoms.

She generally felt anxious, was easily startled and had vivid dreams (all due to poor heart function). She had a weak low back, poor short term memory, mild hay fever in recent years and low libido (due to poor kidney function). Her emotions were variable, she felt a lump in her throat when stressed, and suffered period cramps, clots in her menstrual blood, and usually one week of PMS, feeling irritable, moody and more anxious (all due to stagnated liver function). She had a poor appetite, felt tired and bloated after eating, had food intolerances, was easily bruised, was always thinking and often humming or singing to herself (all related to poor pancreas function). Her energy became very low at three p.m., she suffered lots of colds each year, felt the cold a lot, had sensitive skin and dry hands (due to poor lung function).

Over the first few treatments all these symptoms gradually improved; she eventually felt calm and had a good appetite and energy. After six weeks, she split up with her boyfriend (of two years); her mood remained stable and she coped well with the split up. This is a common pattern with acupuncture treatments. After a few sessions, patients often tell me of big changes in their lives. It seems the treatment enables people to clarify issues in their lives and provides them with the courage to make positive changes.

This patient continued coming for maintenance treatments for years (sometimes once a month, sometimes every few months), through which time she continuously thrived, despite the stresses of a professional career. Her periods became symptom free; she was clear of hay fever, had good memory, concentration, sleep, energy, and had no low back problems.

Energy, sleep, and help to give up smoking

Male, aged 56. This patient initially sought treatment to help him give up smoking and to improve his energy and sleep. He was divorced twenty years ago and now lived alone. He had a stressful job and smoked to relieve the stress.

He also had a small appetite, felt tired after eating, had a poor sense of taste, sweet cravings, tended to worry and think a lot, found it hard to think after midday, and his stools were usually soft or runny (all due to poor pancreas function). His nose ran all day, was worse in the morning but became blocked at night; he was wheezy, for years had felt very sleepy between three and four p.m., was made very tired if he talked a lot, had dry skin, felt the cold, and suffered three to four colds a year (all due to poor lung function). He had palpitations, was easily startled, found it hard to get to sleep, but once asleep had vivid dreams two or three times a week (due to poor heart function). He was hard of hearing in his right ear, had frequent and urgent urination, shortness of breath, poor short term memory when stressed, and felt hot at night (due to poor kidney function). His moods swung high and low and he had dry eyes and high pitch tinnitus (due to stagnated liver function).

It was clear that his poor energy was due to the weakness in the function of both his pancreas and lungs. And he had clearly been driving himself hard for years, which had weakened his kidney function.

By the fifth treatment, his energy was normal (he no longer felt sleepy in the afternoon, nor at any other time of day), his stools were normal, he had no sweet cravings, his nose no longer ran, and he had cut down greatly on the amount he smoked each day. And after a few further treatments he stopped smoking, now regarded himself as a non-smoker and hated the smell of tobacco smoke; his sleep was greatly improved and he often slept solidly; the palpitations had stopped; his sinuses felt clear, and the morning cough which he developed as he started to give up smoking was also greatly improving.

Throat pulsations and general stress

Female, aged 29. This patient initially came for treatment concerning serious throat pulsations, whose cause could not be diagnosed. Her parents were in their late forties when she was conceived and both drove themselves very hard and were exhausted at that time. When born, the patient was deaf in her right ear and had only partial hearing in her left. She now had a stiff low back, frequent and urgent urination, and suffered hay fever for the past two years. She was in a very stressful job and often ran on adrenaline.

These symptoms were all caused by poor kidney function, which she inherited from her parents. This was at the root of her health problems and was exacerbated by her stressful lifestyle. But by this stage in her life, her pancreas, liver and heart were also affected. She had a small appetite, sweet cravings, felt bloated after eating and had excess gas (all due to poor pancreas function). Her emotions were up and down, she had pain on her front and back at the level of her liver, frequent cramps in her calves and feet, sighed a lot, felt a constant lump in her throat, and had painful and heavy periods with one week of PMS, in which she felt frustrated and emotional and had tender and swollen breasts (all due to stagnated liver function). She also had palpitations (due to poor heart function).

Over the first few treatments, all her symptoms (apart from her poor hearing) improved, including the throat pulsations; she said everyone was commenting on how transformed she was. She had taken the contraceptive pill for twelve years and decided to stop. This, combined with the continuing acupuncture treatments, produced a further dramatic improvement in her health (in my experience the contraceptive pill usually weakens the "kidney" function, and stopping this accelerated her improvement).

When taking this patient's heart pulse in one session, I felt a constriction around my throat, and the patient told me that as soon as my finger touched her wrist, her throat started pulsing. This appeared to confirm that her throat pulsations were produced by her heart (which is very often affected by poor kidney function). However, in Chinese medicine, we would normally associate throat-related symptoms with stagnated liver function (which is always exacerbated by stress, if not *caused* by it), so that there appeared to be no clear-cut anatomical explanation for the symptom—beyond my insight that the heart produced it. All that could be concluded was that when the function of her main organs was normalized with acupuncture, the symptom stopped, therefore it must have been the improper function of one or more of those organs that caused it.

Neck pain caused by emotional factors

Female, aged 28. This patient sought treatment for a shoulder and neck pain. She had always had tension and tenderness in her neck, but in the last two to three months it became much worse and she was now getting shooting pains.

She also had food intolerances (to wheat and dairy), felt bloated after eating, with excess gas; her stools were soft and sometimes runny with undigested food in them; she was always thinking and could not accept compliments—in other words, was mentally reluctant to nourish herself (all related to poor pancreas function). She had a poor short term memory, asthma as a child and she used to get hay fever (which stopped two years ago) but was still allergic to cat fur; she felt hot at night; her back was stiff in the mornings; she had weak knees and stiff hips, frequent and urgent urination, shortness of breath when running up stairs, was hard of hearing, and recently felt fearful (all due to poor kidney function). She recently had vivid dreams and was easily startled (due to poor heart function). She was usually emotional and sensitive and tended to feel low, sighed often, recently had mild dizziness, had dry and itchy eyes and saw floaters (which in her case were light, transparent shapes); her menstrual cycle had a variable length, between 33-35 days, with seven days of PMS in which she felt irritable, depressed, angry, and had swollen and tender breasts; and her menstrual blood was dark with clots (all due to stagnated liver function).

This young patient had pronounced poor kidney function, which she clearly inherited from her parents (since she had asthma and hay fever as a child), and this gave her a weak constitution, which meant that the routine stresses of life affected her more deeply than they would most other people.

However, after the first two sessions her neck and shoulder were fine and she felt great, but her neck pain then returned and she started going through emotional turmoil. After the fifth treatment she told me she had a long talk with her boyfriend about many issues and felt much better; she also started "observing herself" at work and managed to relax when she became upset. Her digestion and sleep were now much better, though her energy was still low. For the next two weeks her neck pain got worse again and she said she noticed she was always analysing things and worrying about her insecurities with her boyfriend. The following week she felt good after the treatment, felt more clear and positive and was thinking less; she spoke to her boyfriend about the issues, which improved things; and her neck pain cleared. Her "inner turmoil" was much less and also less intense. The following week, she broke up with her boyfriend. For two weeks after this, her emotions and digestion were up and down but she was feeling much more clear. Her neck and shoulder pain then cleared and generally she felt good; her digestion was good and she started meditation.

This case is a clear illustration of how our physical problems are often directly caused by mental and emotional factors. Her neck pain and digestive problems initially cleared and she felt euphoric after the first session, but then the problems returned since the problems in her relationship with her boyfriend were all unchanged.

Problems with the people or situations in our life can often result in us experiencing a pain in the neck, which is certainly the origin of the expression "pain in the neck". Such pains are usually produced by stagnated liver function, which in this instance was made very much worse by the problem in the patient's life which she could not resolve. This amounted to an obstruction to the flow of her thoughts, which caused stagnated liver function, which then caused the strong pain and stiffness in the gallbladder meridian at her neck and shoulder. It is probably not a coincidence that the gallbladder provides us with the mental ability to make decisions and that our inability to make this type of decision results in dysfunctional tissue along the gallbladder meridian as it leaves the head (the location of the obstructed thoughts).

But with the current patient, the continuing treatments gave her the confidence to face the problems in her life and deal with them, and once she resolved the problems for good, her health issues were able to clear. This is a familiar pattern; patients often tell me of the positive changes they have made in their lives, or that appear to have happened spontaneously since they started treatments.

There is another common pattern that occurs. Some patients (usually particularly strong willed and principled people) are so entrenched in the particular thought patterns that gave rise to most of their physical symptoms, that they cannot escape them. As they start acupuncture treatment, their symptoms initially improve, but then the symptoms return because the patient resumes their previous mental patterns, which reinforces the particular organ malfunctions that produced their symptoms in the first place.

Migraine

Male, aged 24. This patient had a ten-year history of migraines. They improved for about six months but had recently been much worse. He was working as a newly qualified teacher.

The migraines now only started at work; they tended to start at about three p.m. on the right side of his head (around the gallbladder meridian) with a dull sensation which gradually got stronger. He also felt pain behind his right eye, had blurred vision and nausea, and the right side of his neck and his right shoulder would stiffen. Apart from the migraines, he also sighed and suffered hiccups frequently, had cramps in his left leg, saw floaters (specks of light), had a loud voice and was a very structured and organized person (all due to stagnated liver function). He also had a poor short term memory (which was worse in recent years), tended to have a stiff low back, was slightly hard of hearing, had shortness of breath on exertion, mild hay fever (which he had since childhood) and was allergic to dog fur (all due to poor kidney function). He also had vivid dreams, was easily startled, had anxiety, and a slight speech problem (due to poor heart function). He had a small appetite, felt tired after eating, had food allergies, low energy (at work he "kept going on adrenaline" and was very tired in the evening), had sweet cravings, and was always thinking (all related to poor pancreas function).

By the fourth treatment, his headaches were less frequent and also less severe and did not last as long; he was calmer but still slightly anxious. He continued treatments, but with varying gaps between them. He could sometimes go for weeks with no migraines at all, but when the stress of his work was high this tended to trigger a migraine. With a treatment every two weeks, he was generally well and able to cope with the stress of his job, even having periods with no symptoms at all, including the digestive and allergy-related symptoms. He had clearly inherited poor kidney function from his parents (since he had hay fever as a child), which left him with poor stamina; on top of this, his work was extremely demanding and even a person with a strong constitution would have struggled to remain totally healthy while doing the job.

This is a dilemma that many people face and must solve in their own way. If your work is so demanding that your body's resources cannot cope, then if you want to remain healthy (or want to *regain* your health), you would need to either support your health with a system like Chinese acupuncture, change your work, or change the way you respond to your work. The advantage of acupuncture treatment is that it often clarifies all these issues for each person which then enables them to pick the path that is right for them.

Energy, focus, and direction in life

Male, aged 57. This patient sought treatment to improve his energy and "focus" (his sense of direction in life). He ran his own business and previously had two operations on his lower back (fifteen and eight years ago); his discs lumbar-4 and lumbar-5 had "broken up", as he put it. He now experienced back ache and shooting pains down his leg.

In holistic medicine, it is recognised that patients who do not feel supported will often develop a low back problem. In this case, he was used to running a business as a sole trader, and (when viewed metaphorically) his low back vertebra having "broken up" (as he described it) could be likened to the foundations of a bridge crumbling under the strain—the strain of him single-handedly holding up the responsibilities he took on. Any fear concerning our long-term survival would impede the kidney function, which, in turn, would account for the weak spine in the region of the kidneys.

As well as the low back problem, he also had shortness of breath on exertion and an allergy to dust (also due to poor kidney function). He was also easily startled, had palpitations, anxiety attacks, a slight stammer, and had very vivid and strange dreams (all due to poor heart function). He had a quiet voice, and his energy was drained when he talked a lot; he usually felt tired each day around two p.m. onwards; he felt at his best in Autumn (when the lungs are the dominant organ); his sinuses usually felt blocked; he would sweat at night but without feeling hot, and he usually felt "distant" or "not connected" and sad (all related to poor lung function). He had low energy generally, lots of gas, his stools were often very loose, he was always thinking, and had sweet cravings (due to poor pancreas function). He sighed frequently (people were always telling him this), got cramps in his legs and often felt irritated or emotional (due to stagnated liver function).

During the week after his first treatment, he felt very well, alert, had some deep sleeps, and he only felt the afternoon energy lag on one day. By the second week, his energy was up and down, but he felt mentally clearer (he said he did not get stuck in "thinking loops" anymore), and he no longer had the feeling of not being connected. And after a few more treatments, he felt very well, his energy was good, he was feeling more positive and focused and slept solidly with very few dreams.

Although this patient clearly had poor kidney function and poor heart function, which produced significant symptoms, it seems most likely he developed these over a long period of driving himself too hard in life. However, it was clear to me (as a healer) that his personality was dominated by his lungs, and this lung-dominance would have therefore existed *prior* to this. This would have made him a perfectionist, and it was probably this that caused him to drive himself so hard which, in the long run, caused all the other problems.

Abdominal pain and digestive signs

Male, aged 14. The patient's parents split up when he was aged ten, and a year later he developed stomach cramps. His elder brother then left home to attend university, which he also found hard to accept. His stomach cramps persisted for a further two years, when he was brought for treatment.

The pains were almost continuous but were very bad for about two days out of every two weeks. Over the previous two years he was taken to a range of medical practitioners, prescribed an anti-spasmodic drug (*dicyclomine*) which had no effect, and no reason could be found for the pain. The pain consisted mainly of an aching sensation on the centre of his abdomen between the acupoints Ren-8 and Ren-14, sometimes accompanied by stabbing pains at Stomach-25, and the pain was usually worse between seven and eight a.m. and between six and twelve p.m. (these morning hours being when the stomach function was at its strongest and the pericardium at its weakest; and the evening hours being when the large intestine, stomach and pancreas function were at their weakest). These pains had come to dominate his life and led to his exclusion from many activities.

The acupoints the pains were located on clearly indicated poor function of the stomach, large intestine and heart*, and suggested a clear emotional cause in the split up of his parents—he had difficulty stomaching the situation (that is, he could not even *begin* to digest it), which impeded his stomach function; he had difficulty mentally *sorting the good from the bad and letting go of the waste*, which impeded his large intestine function; and his deeply felt social connections had been broken, which impeded his heart function.

He also had a poor appetite, frequent loose stools, felt bloated and tired after eating, but his general energy was ok (all due to poor pancreas function). He often experienced a lump in his throat at night, around eleven p.m., and a strong headache on his temples about four times a week, which usu-

---

* The acupoints Ren-12, Ren-14 and Stomach-25 are the most powerful acupoints on the front of the body associated with the stomach, heart and large intestine respectively.

ally started between six and seven p.m. (due to stagnated liver function). He had hay fever, a stiff low back in the mornings, weak knees which ached after sport, dizziness, and his head usually felt empty after he experienced the pain centred on the acupoint Ren-14, all due to poor kidney function. He experienced vivid dreams about four times a week, and "palpitations" (the pain centred on Ren-14), due to poor heart function. It should be noted that the heart and kidney function are very closely coordinated, which may explain why he felt empty headed (a kidney-related sign) after experiencing the pain on Ren-14, which is a strong heart-related acupoint.

After the first treatment, his mother said he seemed different, had more energy, more "spark", and the abdominal pains were much less for a few days. After a few more treatments his appetite had improved, his stools were variable, but the aching that was centred on Ren-12 was still there each morning and evening. He had weekly treatments over the following four months, with all his symptoms gradually improving, and even being completely absent from time to time. By the end of this course of treatments, he only experienced the pain occasionally, very mildly and for a short time. His energy was good and he was fully engaged in life and (in the words of his mother) was now a healthy thriving teenager.

A classic illustration of Liver invading stomach

At one point in this course of treatments, he felt strong cramping pains at Ren-12 for a few days, with loose stools, and felt tired and sick. His mother said he always felt bad at the start of May, and two of his family members said he often seemed "green around the gills" in this period. It was mid-Spring, which is the time of year that the liver function is at its strongest. And his liver function was also stagnated, his stomach function was weak, and also, *all* his pulses were very "wiry" (indicating that the function of *all* his organs were stagnated due to the influence of his stagnated liver function).

His particular pain and the other signs and symptoms were a graphic, textbook illustration of the Chinese medicine syndrome of "Liver invading stomach" (where his liver stagnation impeded the function of his stomach). But what I found most striking was that his family noticed his green hue, since it was so strong. Green is the colour associated with the liver. The hues on a person's face can often be used diagnostically. Without knowing it, his family had thus diagnosed that his stomach pain was caused by his liver and was due to "Liver invading stomach".

An element of stagnated liver function may also have been caused, or contributed to, by the original emotional traumas in this case. He was clearly a sensitive boy and the loss of his parents and cherished brother, perhaps together with the loss of his previous life (since his pains excluded him from much of that) may have been interpreted by him as the breaking of rules (it was "not fair" that all this was happening to him), which would have obstructed his liver function. Hence, this case also serves as a further demonstration of the interdependence of the organs when processing our thoughts.

Menstrual issues, acne, digestive problems and thrush

Female, aged 32. This patient sought treatment for issues related to her menstrual cycle—primarily acne but also PMS and painful periods; and she also had recurring thrush. For two to three years she was taking an antibiotic acne medication (*tetracycline*) which she also wanted to stop using.

Her menstrual cycle was 35 days long with one week of PMS, in which the acne around her jaw would flare up, and she was also anxious, moody, emotionally up and down and had tender and swollen breasts. On day one of her period she experienced painful cramps with a heavy flow of dark blood with clots (all due to stagnated liver function). One week after her period ended she would experience burning on urination and itching (thrush). She also had a small appetite, felt bloated after eating, had food intolerances, excess gas, loose stools which were sometimes runny and she was always thinking (due to poor pancreas function). Her energy lagged between four and five p.m., she felt the cold, had patches of dry skin, and used her voice heavily in her work (all related to poor lung function). She had poor short term memory, mild hay fever since the age of 21, felt hot at night, was generally very thirsty, and had a frequent headache on her occiput (due to poor kidney function).

She stopped taking the medication immediately and there was a mild flare up of her acne, which is to be expected when any such medication is stopped. However, the flare up was a lot less severe than she anticipated. By the fourth treatment, she had a period and the thrush symptoms were now completely clear and did not return. And after three further months of fortnightly treatments, she was generally feeling well, her digestion was greatly improved, her menstrual cycle had now reverted to 30 days, her period-related symptoms were all reduced, and her acne was greatly improved and not really an issue any more.

Damp heat, and Liver invading the stomach

She was taking the antibiotic for two to three years. Antibiotics deplete the pancreas function. In Chinese medicine terms, this probably contributed to her thrush symptoms, which were *damp heat* in the bladder, the *dampness* being exacerbated by the depleting effect on her pancreas function of the antibiotic. The acne appeared along the stomach meridian on her face and neck and reflected "Stomach heat", which was probably being produced by the stagnated liver function (since each flare up of acne coincided with her PMS phase). The stagnated liver function caused her liver to fail to properly regulate the flow of energy to the stomach, exacerbating the already poor stomach function, which produced the

"Stomach heat". In other words the liver "invaded" the stomach.

Migraines, IBS, sleep, anxiety

Male, aged 49. This patient had a suspected heart attack four months prior to treatment. He was found to have a swollen pericardium (*pericarditis*). He had smoked for many years but immediately gave up when he went into hospital. He worked in a stressful, competitive environment and after a hard day at work, he used to work hard at the gym to help get rid of the stress. He sought acupuncture treatment to address his IBS, migraines, sleep, and stress.

He had a small appetite, poor sense of taste, felt tired and bloated after eating, had loose stools, sweet cravings, and was always thinking (due to poor pancreas function). He usually had blocked sinuses, suffered frequent colds, a sharp energy lag between two and three p.m., was a perfectionist, tended to bear grudges for a long time and found it hard to "let go of things" (all related to poor lung function).

He suffered migraines since childhood. They usually started with very specific visual disturbances, which cleared for about thirty minutes, then the headache started and lasted for about two days. The pain was centred on the temples, was often a dull, background pain but could become intense. This was sometimes accompanied by nausea, a feeling of being detached, and a sensation of pins and needles or numbness in his fingers. He got the migraines about once every two months. When he worked a lot and was very tired, particularly after a period of stress, this usually triggered a migraine. Apart from his migraines, his emotions were unstable, with frequent irritability; he described himself as a control freak with a dislike of impolite people, and of rules being broken (all related to stagnated liver function).

He had vivid dreams for the last ten years and would often shout and jump out of bed in his sleep; he used to suffer frequent panic attacks about twenty years ago, which started again after his father died a few years ago (all these symptoms being due to poor heart function).

He suffered insomnia for many years. He could fall asleep ok, but then always woke around four a.m. with his mind thinking "all sorts of rubbish" related to work and other things, and he was unable to get back to sleep. He felt hot at night, had poor short term memory, poor concentration, an urgent need to urinate when he woke around four a.m.; his ears were often congested, and he had been running on adrenaline for years (all related to poor kidney function).

After the first treatment he felt calmer, had more energy, and did not need to urinate when he woke in the mornings. After the second treatment his concentration was better and he no longer felt the energy lag in the afternoon. After a few more weekly treatments his IBS symptoms had cleared, he was "not worrying about stuff", no longer felt hot at night and slept solidly. He continued to have regular treatments, at two or three weekly intervals, and only had an occasional migraine, which was usually less severe than previously—he often experienced the same visual disturbances but these did not usually develop into the migraine. He was a "driven" person who continued to work and play hard, and the regular treatments were required to counter the depleting effects of this, particularly on his kidney function.

Jaw pain caused by life issues the patient could not stomach

This patient was clearly a very sensitive person. In the second treatment session, he also told me about a deep aching pain around his jaw which he had for about two years. I asked if there was any situation in his life over this time that he could not stomach. He described a serious conflict with his neighbour which had built up for years; recently it progressed to the stage where he physically assaulted the neighbour.

Every other neighbour had similar problems with this same person. The problem was so bad, the patient considered moving house. Along with addressing the other issues mentioned above, I also treated the jaw pain directly, needling the acupoints Stomach-6 and Stomach-12, which was also tender. The jaw pain cleared immediately and did not return. As mentioned above, he felt calmer and said he did not let things bother him anymore. It was clear that this jaw pain, on the stomach meridian, was caused by the fact that he could not stomach the situation in his life. In other words, his mental inability to even *begin* digesting the situation impeded his stomach function, which is what produced the pain on the stomach meridian—specifically, as it passed over his jaw. In this way, our body's symptoms are often metaphorical.

Extreme stress and grief

Female, aged 65. When this patient first sought treatment, a close friend of hers had died two days before. She was also retiring from a professional career, and was under great stress due to her son's substance abuse.

She smoked since the age of 16 and had no wish to give up smoking, only saying that she felt a bit croaky in the mornings. She also had shadows under her eyes from her late forties, had weak knees, tended to get achy knees and hips in Winter or if walking for about five miles; she had a stiff lumbar region and had problems with her low back for most of her life; she had frequent and urgent urination which started in recent years, very bad short-term memory, was slightly hard of hearing, got headaches at her occiput every two weeks, felt hot at night, thirsty during the day, and experienced hot flushes in the day about once a week, particularly when she was upset or anxious (all due to poor kidney function). When stressed, she felt a "hollow" feeling in her throat, like an uncomfortable space; she was irritable, got low when she worried about things (she felt she "could not cope with what the world was throwing at her"); she would often wake with a pain behind her eyes; she got cramp in her toes, and her nails had ridges. Her periods stopped at age fifty, but before this she would get PMS for three to four days and had bad pains on day one of her period (all related to stagnated liver function). She had palpitations, was easily startled, which started when her son was having drug and alcohol problems (due to poor heart function*). She felt the cold, which had always been the same, would get sneezing fits, and her energy was low in the afternoon (due to poor lung function).

After her first treatment, she initially felt very tired, which lasted for two days, but following this she felt greatly energized and positive. In the weeks that followed, she described herself as being under a lot of strain related to problems with her son, but was coping well with the stress and was sleeping well. She was feeling calmer, and found it easier to emotionally detach herself from the problems with her son, and was thinking clearly. After three months of fortnightly treatments, her hot flushes had cleared, the eye shadows greatly improved, and her low back felt better. Six weeks later, her son died of an overdose. After a few weekly treatments, she was coping well with her loss and increased the interval between treatments to one month.

Wrist pain due to a previous bereavement

About one year later, having mainly recovered from her loss, she developed a pain in her left wrist, along the lung meridian. There was no injury and the pain appeared to start spontaneously. When I told her my diagnosis (that this represented the emotional pain related to her bereavement, which her lungs were now recovering from), this made perfect sense to

* It is significant that her heart function was clearly impeded due to the difficulties in her emotional connections, which highlights the mental/emotional functions of the heart, and how difficulties in these areas can physically weaken the heart.

her. She told me she had been cradling her wrist in the last few days, like you would a baby.

Panic attacks and hay fever

Male, aged 45. This patient sought treatment for panic attacks. His father died three months previously and since then he suffered panic attacks, which were usually triggered by stress at work.

He had palpitations (awareness of his heartbeat), vivid dreams and nightmares, anxiety (which triggered nausea and pins and needles in his hands), panic attacks, after which he felt lightheaded (all due to poor heart function). He also had hay fever, which he had since childhood, with sinus pain, a runny nose, tightness in the chest and itching in his throat; he was allergic to dust and animal fur, had poor short term memory (which had always been the same), was hot at night, and heard a low pitch buzzing sound during the panic attacks (all due to poor kidney function).

It transpired that the patient's father was aged 48 when the patient was conceived, which probably explains why the patient was born with poor kidney function.

He also felt bloated after eating, had loose stools; his head felt muzzy each morning, but cleared after he was up for an hour or so—which had also always been the same; he had sweet cravings and was always thinking (all related to poor pancreas function). He had heartburn about once a week, which he felt as a hot sensation rising up the centre of his chest (due to poor stomach function). He was also quickly irritated, with fluctuating emotions, often got depressed, felt a lump in his throat, had cramp in his feet about twice a month (on the liver meridian), frequently had red and dry eyes; had frequent headaches on the temples and behind the eyes and at night had visual disturbances (all due to stagnated liver function).

All his symptoms gradually improved over the first seven weekly treatments, and by that time he had no hay fever symptoms whatsoever, despite it being hay fever season. The previous year, his hay fever symptoms were the worse they had ever been and he said the acupuncture treatment seemed like a miracle cure. After one of the early treatments, he returned the following week and told me his sinuses were clear and his sense of smell was dramatically improved; he was now noticing the smells everywhere which he was previously unaware of and complained of the world seeming almost *too* smelly.

His digestive signs were all improved (including his muzzy head in the morning, which was now gone completely); his energy was good; he was sleeping well with only an occasional dream, and had no nightmares; he felt calm and his anxiety was only mild and occasional.

He continued treatment, gradually increasing the interval between treatments from three weeks to six weeks. He clearly inherited poor kidney function from his parents (since he had hay fever from childhood), which left him with a weak constitution, but the monthly acupuncture treatments enabled him to cope with the stresses of life and remain healthy and largely symptom free. He now ran his own successful business which he set up a few weeks after starting the acupuncture treatments. This, as I have said elsewhere, is a very familiar pattern—after a few weeks of starting the treatments, patients often tell me of big changes they have made in their lives, or of significant opportunities that appear to have spontaneously come their way.

As with the previous case history, this case also serves as a clear illustration of the effect on the heart of emotional factors. The patient already had lifelong poor kidney function, and when his father died, the break in this strong social connection impeded his heart function, which caused his panic attacks (a heart-related symptom). Incidentally, if he had not also had the underlying poor kidney function, the impediment to his heart function would probably not have been sufficient to produce the panic attacks. But since his kidney function was already poor, this lessened the "stamina" of his heart—due to the "six channel theory" association between the heart and kidney.

Hernia treated with acupuncture

Male, aged 34. This patient initially sought treatment for a pain in his neck and shoulder, and a frequent lumbar pain. He also had a long history of hay fever, starting in childhood, and had other clear signs of poor kidney function (shortness of breath when running up stairs, wheezing when exercising, poor hearing in one ear, feeling hot at night). He ran his own business and was a sporty person.

After the initial treatments, which cleared all his significant symptoms, he came for routine maintenance treatments every month or two, for a period of around six years.

About two years after he started treatments with me, he reported feeling a "hernia" type pain, which had been developing for a few weeks. He thought it started due to an injury while canoeing. The pain was on the right of his abdomen, at the acupoint Stomach-26, and the pain radiated down the inside of his leg, on the liver meridian.

Apart from acupoints for his general treatment, I also needled Stomach-26.

Four weeks later he returned for another routine maintenance treatment. The hernia pain was still a problem. When getting out of bed in the morning, he felt a stabbing pain; and when canoeing, he felt a shooting pain.

Apart from general constitutional acupoints, I also needled *ashi* points on his right side, from Stomach-26 downwards, and also three acupoints on the liver meridian, Liver-12 to Liver-10.

Three weeks later he returned. The hernia pain was completely clear for a few days after the last treatment. The following week he went canoeing, and experienced no pain, but over the following few days, the pain returned and got worse; and he described himself as being in agony. He consulted his doctor, who said she could feel a tear in the muscle, so she referred him to a specialist at the hospital for surgery. But the initial consultation with the surgeon was three to four weeks away. He then had another canoeing session and there was no hernia pain during the session, but he still felt the pain every morning when getting out of bed. He asked if I could focus on treating the hernia, since, even if there was only a chance I could heal it before he saw the surgeon, then he could avoid having surgery.

I needled the same acupoints as in the previous treatment, only this time I added moxibustion as well.

One week later he returned. The day after the last treatment the hernia pain was worse, and was now worse along the whole line, from around Stomach-26 down to Liver-10. He had avoided canoeing this week.

I repeated the previous treatment.

Six days later he returned. This time, the pain was not worse after the previous treatment; and he now felt a dull ache around Liver-10 to Liver-11, and a stabbing pain at Stomach-26. Again, he had avoided canoeing.

I needled *ashi* points again, but the locations had moved slightly. I needled four acupoints near to Stomach-26, and two acupoints about two *cun* below Liver-10.

Three weeks later he returned. Since the last treatment, he did one whole day of canoeing, and afterwards a bruise developed near to Stomach-26 which was the size of a tennis ball and he felt sick and bloated. He attended his appointment at the hospital, and the surgeon performed an ultrasound scan. The surgeon reported that at the exact location where the hernia was, there was a slight bulge in the muscle, as if a previous injury had healed. But otherwise, there was no problem and he was discharged. Since then, the patient had not experienced the hernia pain, though there was a slight ache in that same location.

In this session, I only treated him constitutionally and avoided using any of the acupoints related to the previous hernia treatments.

Three weeks later he returned for a routine maintenance treatment. The hernia was now completely clear and remained so for the following few years that I treated him.

The findings of the patient's doctor and also the surgeon provided compelling evidence that the acupuncture had healed this patient's hernia. However, even more compelling evidence would have been provided if an ultrasound scan had been performed *before* my treatments, as well as after, since there was only the experience of the patient's family doctor to confirm that a hernia was definitely present before my treatments. The patient confirmed he had never experienced a hernia before in that location and had certainly never had surgery there. But I suspect that even if an ultrasound scan *had* been performed before my treatments, sceptics would still choose to disbelieve the treatment outcome, simply claiming that the hernia must have got better by itself. And to be fair to the sceptics, when there is nothing in their own knowledge that could possibly account for the treatment outcome, what other choices would be open to them?

Note on the general "symptom picture" of a patient

None of the above patients were taking strong pharmaceutical remedies, hence their "symptom picture" was clear and made perfect sense from the Chinese medicine point of view—and their response to treatment was exactly as expected. I deliberately selected such case studies since this best illustrates the effects of Chinese acupuncture. With these patients, their main organs functioned (and also malfunctioned) just as human organs had always done; and the patterns of organ malfunction identified by Chinese physicians over the last two thousand years were clearly identifiable in these patients today.

When I take the case history of a new patient and they describe their symptoms, it quickly becomes obvious whether or not a patient is taking strong pharmaceutical remedies. With those that *are*, their symptoms fail to make sense, and certainly do not fall into any of these historical Chinese medicine patterns of organ malfunction. Yet with those who are *not* taking such remedies, their symptom picture always makes perfect sense. In fact, sometimes I have wondered if such patients had read a textbook on Chinese medicine and were simply reciting the symptoms from a list they had read. Of course they were not doing this. But the nature and pattern of their symptoms were often so textbook "Chinese medicine" that it was uncanny.

The chemistry of the body is extremely complex and changes from second to second. All the organs send chemical messages through the blood to coordinate their function with that of the other organs and systems in the body. However, most strong pharmaceutical remedies are designed to attempt to take control of a particular aspect of the body's chemistry. And since the normal function of the organs relies on their ability to constantly vary the complex chemistry of the body, any measures that diminish the chemical autonomy of the organs will, inevitably, ultimately prevent the organs from functioning as nature intended. Hence, the symptoms and patterns of malfunction which have been present through history, no longer occur, so that the symptom picture is muddled and makes little sense when compared to the patterns identified by Chinese medicine (as relayed in this book).

Treating such patients is often challenging. Sometimes only small improvements are possible, which may only last for a day or two before the undesirable symptoms reappear. When the body no longer enjoys its chemical autonomy, this also tends to prevent natural healing systems like Chinese acupuncture from working. Such systems achieve their results by using some natural method to prompt the organs to resume their normal function. The healing therefore relies on the body's command of its own chemistry to effect the healing, but because the organs no longer have chemical autonomy, they cannot make the necessary adjustments—at least not permanently. However, acupuncture can still be used to give temporary relief from the undesirable effects of such remedies. And further, acupuncture is probably one of the most effective systems for providing this relief, since it corrects organ malfunction directly, without attempting to interact with the chemical or hormonal control systems—the very systems that pharmaceutical remedies act upon. This last fact probably also explains why such relief is only temporary—the organ functions are initially normalized by acupuncture, but they adopt the same malfunctions again, since the organs no longer have chemical autonomy and so cannot sustain normal function.

Further reading

This book is a reduction of a much larger book by the same author:

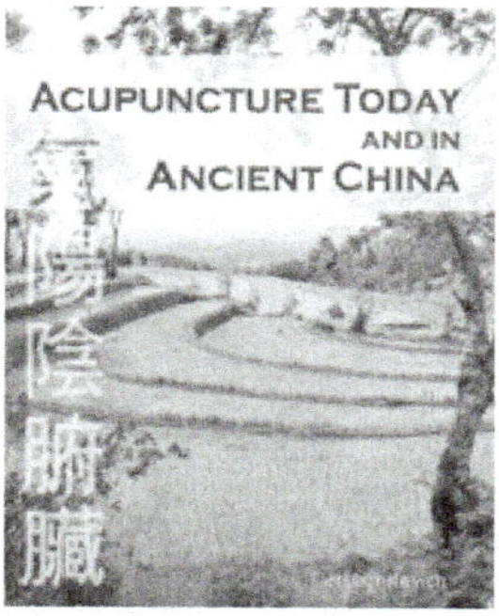

Acupuncture Today and in Ancient China provides much greater detail on

- the history of Chinese medicine;
- the development of its theories of metabolism;
- the organ functions, which are explained at length and compared to those described in contemporary physiology;
- the translation between *Nei Jing* concepts and those of contemporary physiology;
- much greater detail concerning the mental functions of the organs;
- a detailed analysis of key *Nei Jing* concepts, such as Five phase theory, the notion of *chi*, and terms such as kidney *jing*;

- references to the *Nei Jing* texts where each of the organ signs or symptoms were first mentioned; and
- much detail on the scientific investigations into what acupuncture is and how it works, including the author's own cutting-edge research into how acupuncture works.

Free sample chapters can also be downloaded in pdf format, from **www.curiouspages.com/atac**

Index of signs, symptoms, and conditions

Made in the USA
Monee, IL
04 November 2026

67379473R00089